The Recipe for Radiance

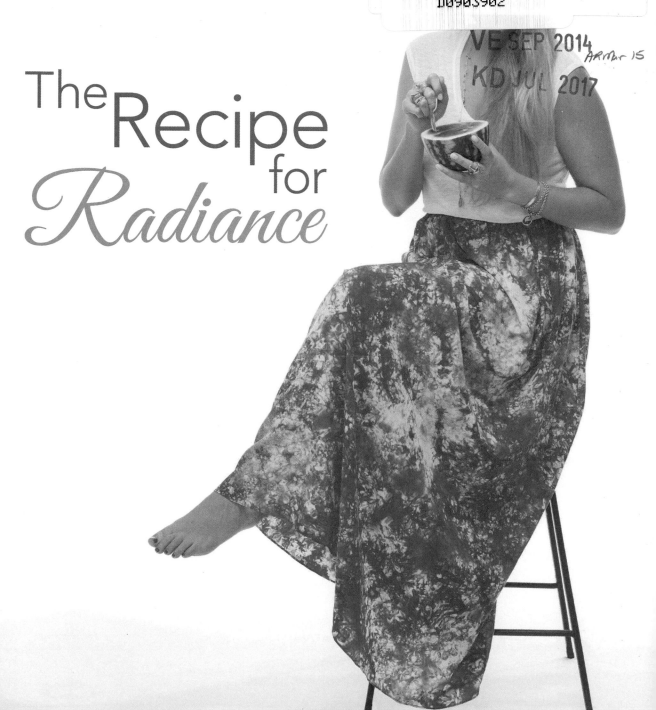

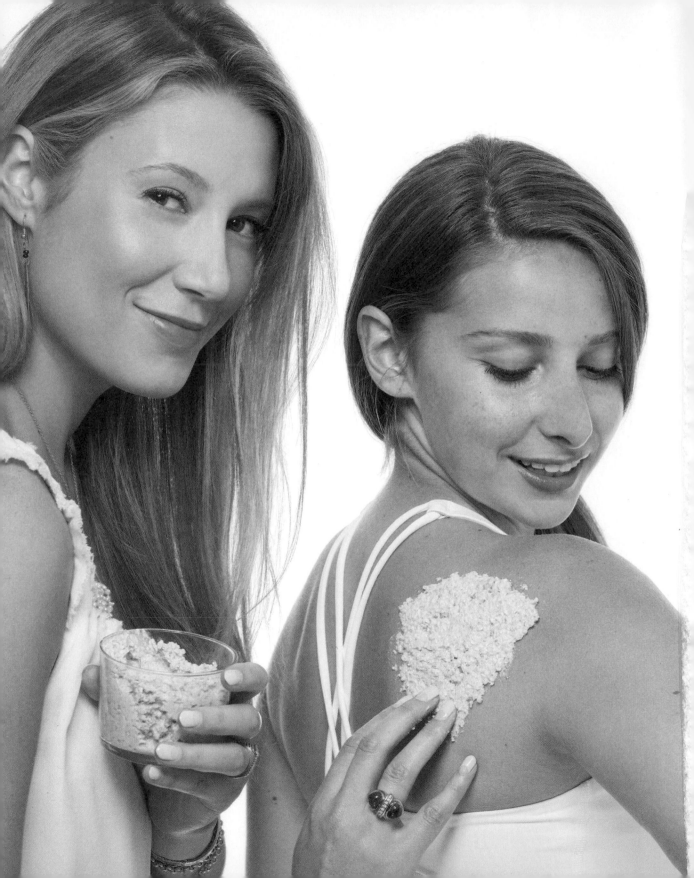

The Recipe for Radiance

Discover Beauty's Best-Kept Secrets in Your Kitchen

Alexis Wolfer

Photography by Evan Sung

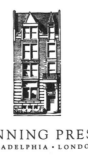

Running Press
PHILADELPHIA · LONDON

© 2014 by Alexis Wolfer
Photography © 2014 by Evan Sung
Published by Running Press,
A Member of the Perseus Books Group

Printed in China

Books published by Running Press are available at special
discounts for bulk purchases in the United States by
corporations, institutions, and other organizations. For more
information, please contact the Special Markets Department
at the Perseus Books Group, 2300 Chestnut Street, Suite 200,
Philadelphia, PA 19103, or call (800) 810-4145, ext. 5000,
or e-mail special.markets@perseusbooks.com.

ISBN 978-0-7624-5040-4
Library of Congress Control Number: 2013953426

E-book ISBN 978-0-7624-5186-9

9 8 7 6 5 4 3 2
Digit on the right indicates the number of this printing

Edited by Cindy De La Hoz
Designed by Corinda Cook

Photography: Evan Sung
Photography assistant: Eric Bissell

Food styling: Suzanne Lenzer
Food styling assistant: Ashely Schleeper

Prop styling: Maeve Sheridan
Prop styling assistant: Kristen Usui

Hair and makeup: Desirae Cherman

Models: Abeba Davis, Jeanette Eng, Sharlotta Kay, Katelyn
O'Friel, Annika Sundin, Carly Wolfer

Typography: Avenir, Gotham, Great Vibes, Lomba,
and Melbourne

Running Press Book Publishers
2300 Chestnut Street
Philadelphia, PA 19103-4371

Visit us on the web!
www.runningpress.com
www.offthemenublog.com

Dedication

For all of the women and girls out there who think they're anything less than stunningly gorgeous, know this: you are beautiful exactly as you are. Makeup, skin care, and, yes, even these beauty recipes are fun and glamorous, but they neither determine nor define your beauty. Your *real beauty* exudes from within. Don't let anyone ever tell you otherwise.

In memory of my papa, Dr. James J. Feffer, who taught me the power of education, hard work, and knowledge; and showed me the value of integrity, loyalty, poise, and kindness. Hoping this is "of interest."

Contents

Introduction 13

Guidelines 16

Chapter 1: Face 19

Acne, Breakouts, Pimples, + Zits 20

APPLY

Hydrating + Blemish-Fighting Facial Mask . . . 23

Tropical Fruit Peel 24

Calming + Clearing Milk Mask 24

Anti-Acne Apple Astringent 26

EAT

Orange Sunshine Soup 28

Asian Cabbage Slaw 29

Raw Oatmeal 31

Fine Lines + Wrinkles 32

APPLY

Age-Reversing Wine Mask 34

Strawberry + Champagne Serum 34

Piña Colada Polish 37

EAT

Seared Tuna with Mushroom + Scallion
"Fried" Brown Rice 39

Chilled Thai Almond Butter Noodles 40

Almond Butter + Strawberries 42

Sea Greens Salad 43

Age Spots + Hyperpigmentation 44

APPLY

Pumpkin Key Lime Brightener 46

Geisha's Secret Sake Serum 46

Skin-Lightening Spot Treatment 49

EAT

Nut Butter Chicken Salad Wrap 51

Pumpkin Pie Pancakes + Cranberry
Maple Syrup 52

Green Papaya Salad 54

Sweet Potato Chips + Cumin Dip 55

Redness + Rosacea 56

APPLY

Healing Herbal Tonic 58
Cooling Coffee Compresses 58
Cucumber + Rose Redness Remedy 61

EAT

Mint + Ginger Green Tea Lemonade 64
Pan-Seared Sea Scallops + Truffled Shiitake
  Rice 65
Beet Salad with Fennel, Orange, + Sunflower
  Gremolata 67
Lemon Berry Parfait 68

Dull, Dry, Drab Skin 70

APPLY

Avocado + Oatmeal Revival Mask 72
Sweet Lip Scrub 75
Strawberry + Kiwi Fruit Peel 75
Pumpkin + Coconut Gommage 76

EAT

Tropical Crab Salad 78
Raw Green Soup 78
Wild Strawberries + "Top of the Waldorf
  Rooftop Honey"-Infused Yogurt 80
Protein Crackers with Avocado 81

Chapter 2: Eyes 83

Under-eye Circles 84

APPLY

Perk-Up Potato Packs 86
Egg-cellent Eye Gel 86
Faux-Rested Eye Mask 89
Iced Tea Toner 89

EAT

Garden Vegetable Omelet 91
Coffee Rubbed Chicken + Farro Salad 92
Creamy Kale + Walnut Salad 94

Smile Lines, Crow's Feet, +
Other Eye Wrinkle Euphemisms 95

APPLY

Two-in-One Anti-Aging Makeup Remover . . . 97
Plump 'Em Up Eye Mask 99
Rejuvenating Eye Polish 100

EAT

Dukkah-Honey Crusted Halibut 103
Raw Brownie Batter Pudding 105
Grilled Salmon Salad 105

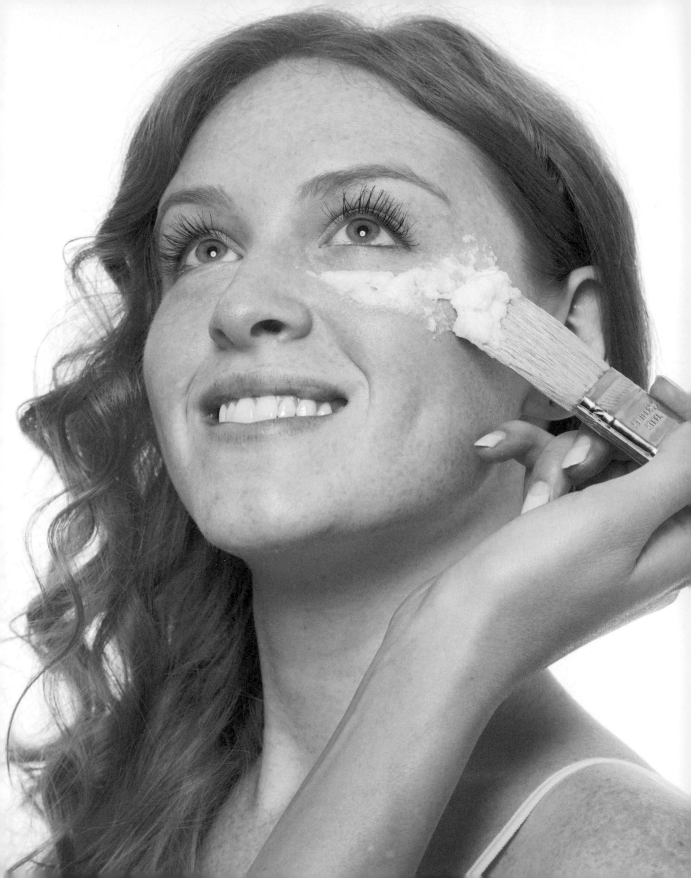

Red, Itchy, Puffy, Bloodshot Eyes 106

APPLY

Optic Tea Treatment 108
Cucumber + Yogurt Cooler 108
Gooseberry Meringue Mask 111

EAT

Cereal Crusted Asparagus Fries + Yogurt
　　Dipping Sauce 114
Honey Glazed Tofu + Orange Broccoli 116
Mexicali Rockfish Ceviche 117

Chapter 3: Body 119

Sunburn 120

APPLY

Sweet Watermelon Serum 122
Milk + Honey Calming Compresses 122
Cooling Cucumber Mask 125
Basil Soothing Spray 125

EAT

Shaved Fennel + Blood Orange Salad 127
Balsamic + Goat Cheese Stuffed Figs 127
Roasted Watermelon Gazpacho 128
Roasted Broccoli + Sun-Dried Tomato
　　Spaghetti 130
Classic Collard Greens 131

Cellulite 132

APPLY

Cellulite-Concealing Coffee Scrub 135
Detoxifying Seaweed Bath 136
Coconut Polish 136

EAT

Raw Creamsicle Milk Shake 139
Creamy Salmon Cucumber Boats 141
Chopped Veggie Spice Salad 142
Mediterranean Turkey Burgers 143

Body Breakouts 144

APPLY

Yogurt + Baking Soda Buffer 146
Strawberry Clearing Mask 146
Starry Spot Treatment 149

EAT

Bocconcino di Tartara 151
Giardino 151
Creamy Butternut Squash Porridge 152

Stretch Marks 154

APPLY

Sweet Potato + Honey Healer 157

Rejuvenating Scar Scrub 157

Ginger + Turmeric Massage Oil 158

EAT

Sweet Green Smoothie 161

Avocado, Watercress, + Cumin Salad 161

Grilled Nut Butter + Apple Sandwich 163

Dry Skin + Rough Patches 164

APPLY

Baby Bottom Balm 167

Creamy Skin Treatment 167

Lemonade Lightening Scrub 169

EAT

Olive Oil Granola 171

Kale Chips + Spicy Cucumber Dip 172

Honey Roasted Delicata Squash Salad 174

Donna Karan's Daily Green Juice 175

Uneven Skin Tone + Texture (+ Self-Tanner Mishaps!) . . . 176

APPLY

Cantaloupe + Carrot Illuminating Mask 179

Margarita Brightening Scrub 180

Lightening Overnight Toner 180

EAT

Charred Red Pepper Dip 183

Portobello Mushroom "Pizza" + Mesclun
    Greens 185

Blueberry Crustless Quiche 186

Grilled Pineapple with Cashew Butter + Vanilla
    Frozen Yogurt 188

Ingrown Hairs + Razor Burn 189

APPLY

Pre-Shave Oil 191

Skin Soothing After Shave 193

Daily Exfoliating Scrub 194

EAT

Tropical Popeye 197

Turmeric Dip 197

Kabocha Squash with Walnut Pesto 199

Fingers + Feet 200

APPLY

Softening Beer Bath 202

Nail-Whitening Soak 202

Out-of-Control Cuticles Cure 205

Hydrating Hand + Foot Mask 206

Callous Removing Scrub 206

EAT

Maple-Glazed Coconut Cashews 208

Vegetarian Pâté 209

Farro + Tuna Salad 210

Chapter 4: Hair 213

Thinning, Fine, Slow-Growing Hair 214

APPLY

Spicy Tequila Scalp Toner 216
Volumizing Hair Rinse 216
Sour Cream Exfoliating Hair Mask 219
Thinning Hair Booster Tonic 219

EAT

Creamless Creamed Spinach 221
Sun-Dried Tomato + Basil Breakfast
   Burrito 222
Three-Bean Salad with Shrimp 224
Balsamic Grilled Salmon + Creamy Cranberry
   Rice 225

Dry, Dull Hair + Scalp 226

APPLY

Farewell Flakes Scalp Mask 229
Take It All Off Clarifying Toner 229
Shine-Enhancing Conditioning Treatment . . 230

EAT

Gingered Wild Salmon with Apple Shallot
   Brandy Glaze 233
Baked Coconut Shrimp + Sweet Potato Mash
   with Spicy Marmalade 235
Vanilla + Cardamom Chia Seed Pudding . . . 237

Frizz + Other Hair Damage 238

APPLY

Strand-Saving Sweet Hair Mayonnaise 240
Strand-Saving Beach Spray 243
Frizz-Fighting Serum 243

EAT

Chinese Five-Spiced Nuts 246
Eggs + Sweet Potato Hash 247
Sardines with Plumped Raisins, Wilted Arugula,
   + Croutons 248

Acknowledgments 250

Index 253

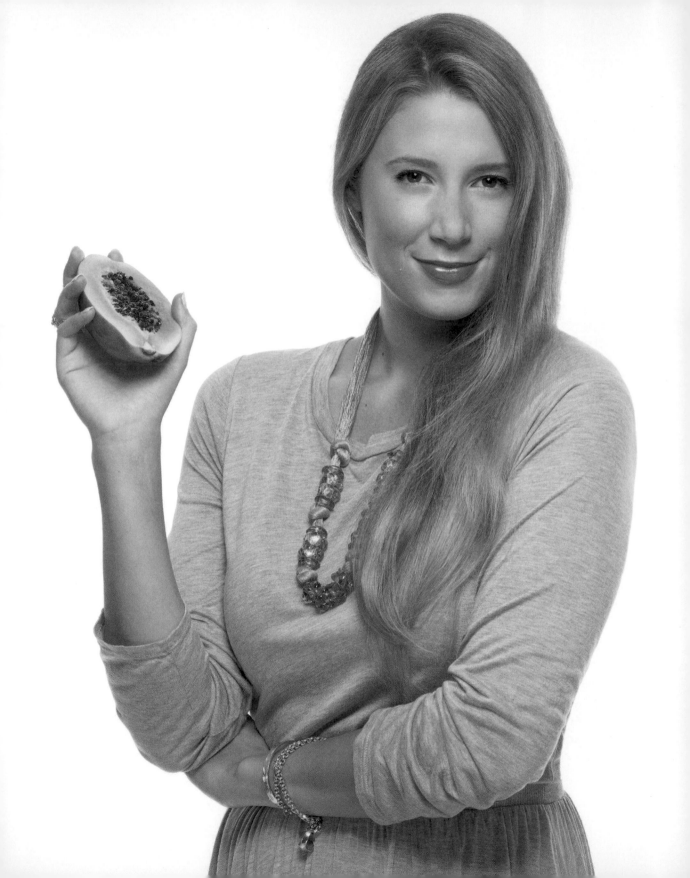

Introduction

So many of us obsess over calories, fat grams, and carbohydrates in the quest for beauty, but we're doing it all wrong. If the goal is to be beautiful (and I don't know a woman for whom that's not the goal!), we need to ditch the low-carb, fat-free, whatever-is-next fad diet and fundamentally shift our perspective. We need to put ourselves on a beauty diet—one that embraces the power of food and its impact on our looks both when eaten and applied topically.

Want to be more beautiful? Say good-bye to diets that may make you drop pounds but leave your complexion dull and hair drab. Wave farewell to all those pricey store-bought products lining your bathroom counters, many of them packed with chemicals, providing questionable results and draining your wallet. Instead, meet me in your kitchen, because that's where you'll find the key to radiant skin, thick hair, and strong nails. You just need to know the recipes—the same ones that led *Access Hollywood* to dub me "Female Beauty MacGyver" and *People StyleWatch* to name me "The DIY Queen"—and now you have them!

I say all this with conviction and confidence now, but I didn't always know that food was the key to beauty.

For a long time, I thought beauty was a number on a scale, a pricey skin cream, and perfectly painted nails. When an eating disorder brought me to that number, Estée Lauder gave me that crème, and a manicure gave me those nails, I realized how wrong I was. Instead of Cindy Crawford-like looks, I had thinning hair, dull skin, and weakened (albeit perfectly polished) nails. My diet—the diet I had so strictly adhered to in the hope of achieving some ever-elusive beauty ideal—was backfiring.

It finally dawned on me, you really are what you eat. (And nobody wants to be sugar-free Jell-O.)

A diet that considered Crystal Light and cucumbers "food groups" had an intensely negative effect on my hair, nails, skin, and eyes. That made me acutely aware of the power of food and the holistic connection between our bodies and our beauty. So, I changed gears. (Well, that's oversimplifying things, but I'll spare you the saga, because who wants the lengthy story when I can just skip right to the juicy parts?) Bottom line: I started to EAT for beauty and the payoff was profound. It fundamentally changed how I approached both my personal beauty regimen as well as my career in the beauty industry.

Combining my professional background in beauty editorial and my master's degree in women's rights, I had already begun to launch TheBeautyBean.com as the ultimate place for women to get their beauty and lifestyle information in a more empowering way. Where most women's magazines were predicated on making women feel crummy about themselves in the hopes of selling them the latest fix, I wanted to help empower women to live more beautiful lives, to subtly promote better body images, and to prevent eating disorders. Merely eliminating the unrealistic beauty ideals promoted in most women's publications in the hope of creating a place where women could get all their desired lifestyle content in a more positive way wasn't enough though.

Once I realized the power food had over our beauty (and it wasn't about eliminating food groups or crash dieting), I had to do more. I had developed a level of expertise that led me to appear on *Today*, share DIY beauty tips with Martha Stewart, and put champagne on a model's face on *E! News*. Now I wanted to share all I knew about feeding your body for beauty, to help women take back the power of food for beauty the same way I had.

When I finally realized that my skin is my body's largest organ, everything else started to make sense and I wanted to share this ultimate beauty secret! How I was feeding my body was how I was feeding my hair, skin, nails, and every other part of me. When you sweat (one of our body's primary detoxifying mechanisms), you push the by-products of your diet through your skin. No wonder I was breaking out from all those artificial sweeteners, and suffering from dry skin on a diet that was pretty much entirely fat-free. My hair and nails were failing to grow in as quickly and strongly as I liked. No shocker there! I was barely consuming any protein, let alone any iron or any of the essential B vitamins required for healthy hair and nails.

Moreover, I realized that if my skin is a means by which my body expels toxins and reflects my health and wellness, it's also a sponge, absorbing everything I put on it. If there was ever a time when my eating disorder proved useful, it was in my delusional fear that if over the course of the month I applied an entire bottle of body lotion, I was absorbing (and, thus, gaining) that weight. While that premise is embarrassing to admit, it made me realize that while my beauty products didn't lead to weight gain, they were most definitely being absorbed by my skin. In the same way that my pores were able to carry toxins out of my body, they were similarly capable of transporting whatever I put on my skin deep within my body.

It became glaringly obvious how many beauty products were coming across my desk at The Beauty Bean that boasted of including the latest fad food as an ingredient. From anti-aging creams packed with coconut oil to anti-acne cleansers ripe with fruit acids, it seemed like every new beauty product on the market was tapping into the beauty benefits found in food. Which, naturally, got me thinking: Why not just go to the source?

I started to feed my body for beauty, topically and internally, with food. I wanted to glow. I wanted skin so clear and smooth it radiated (in a non-oily way). I wanted hair thick and lustrous and strong enough to handle a daily dose of heat styling and a regular dousing of hair dye, without showing the effects. I wanted nails hard as steel. I wanted eyes that smiled and a forehead that frowned, both without lingering lines. I set out to find the secrets and—lots of research and many beauty experiments later—I found them in my kitchen!

And, well, since I've never been one for keeping secrets, now I'm spilling all my favorite beauty-boosting recipes to create both healthy, delicious meals that will promote beauty from the inside out as well as easy, affordable, and all-natural topical beauty treatments to boost your beauty from the outside in.

Ready to get cooking? Read on to discover my favorite recipes that promote beauty from within (did you know a diet rich in kale can reduce under-eye circles?) as well as my top topical DIY beauty recipes (like my coffee scrub that can reduce cellulite!). Don't just trust me; in the pages of this book you'll not only find my own DIY beauty recipes but also secrets shared with me for this book by celebrities, models, chefs, and beauty editors (including Kristin Chenoweth, Brooklyn Decker, Vanessa Williams, Byrdie Bell, Donna Karan, and many, many more)!

Whether you're looking to overhaul your routine, want some all-natural home remedies to add to your beauty arsenal, or just need some ideas for the next time you're in a bind, you've come to the right place! And, no, you don't need to toss all your favorite beauty products. (I most certainly haven't. I am a beauty editor, after all!) But with beauty recipes like these—and results you can see—you may just decide to free up some of that bathroom space your old products once took.

Have a pressing beauty concern? Flip ahead to whatever section of the book speaks to you. Or, start at the beginning and end at the end. Either way, within these pages you will learn both how to APPLY and EAT for beauty, all in your kitchen!

Beautifully,
Alexis

P.S. Have questions? Tweet me @AlexisWolfer

For more tips, visit www.TheBeautyBean.com

Guidelines

I may not believe in beauty rules (hey, if you like that blue lipstick and can rock it confidently, go for it!), but here are a few—mostly common sense—guidelines, for using this book.

1. If you're allergic to any of the ingredients in a recipe, steer clear.

2. If any of the APPLY recipes burn, sting, tingle, itch, or otherwise cause any discomfort whatsoever, rinse them off immediately and seek medical attention if the symptoms persist.

3. Talk with a doctor before starting any new routine—whether it's a new beauty regimen or a diet.

4. Unless a recipe is specifically designed for your eye area, avoid the area immediately around your eyes. The skin around your precious peepers is extraordinarily thin and sensitive and some ingredients aren't safe for use near them.

5. Similarly, if a recipe is designed for your body, do not use it on your face. The skin on your face requires far more care than your body. If, however, you want to use a face recipe on your body, go for it!

6. Do not use any of the APPLY recipes on open skin. That pimple you picked at may be pining for a dose of my Anti-Acne Apple Astringent (page 26), but wait until the skin has healed before going there.

7. When possible, choose organic. If you're going to make your own beauty products or prepare your own meals, you may as well feed your body with the most wholesome ingredients possible. Genetically modified foods and produce doused in pesticides are not nearly as safe as their organic counterparts.

8. When I say "eggs," I mean large, brown, cage-free, and grass-fed ones. Mostly, because I believe that the happier the chicken, the happier the egg—and who doesn't want the happiest of eggs in their recipes?!

9. Since we're working with fresh ingredients, most APPLY recipes should be used immediately or kept in the refrigerator in an airtight container for no longer than three days, unless otherwise specified.

10. Unlike with harsh chemicals that may give faster results—often at the expense of your wellness, health, and wallet—the APPLY recipes here rely on all-natural ingredients. As a result, benefits are cumulative with continued use and may take time to appear. Be patient.

11. Eating for beauty also requires patience. Consider how long it takes for your hair to grow just one inch (usually about two months!). So keep in mind it will take time for these beauty boosting EAT recipes to work their magic. But trust me, when they do, it will all be worth it!

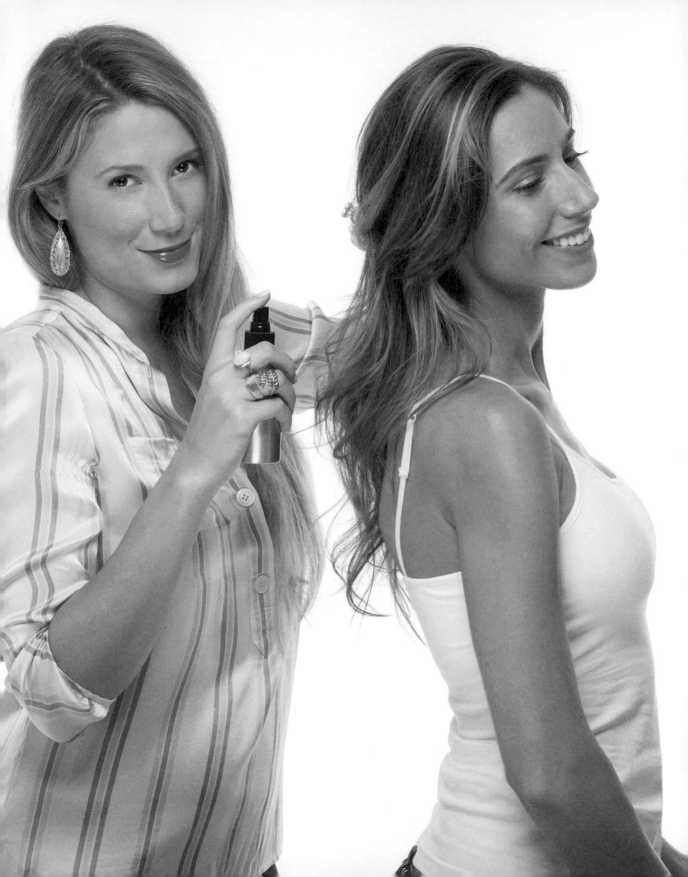

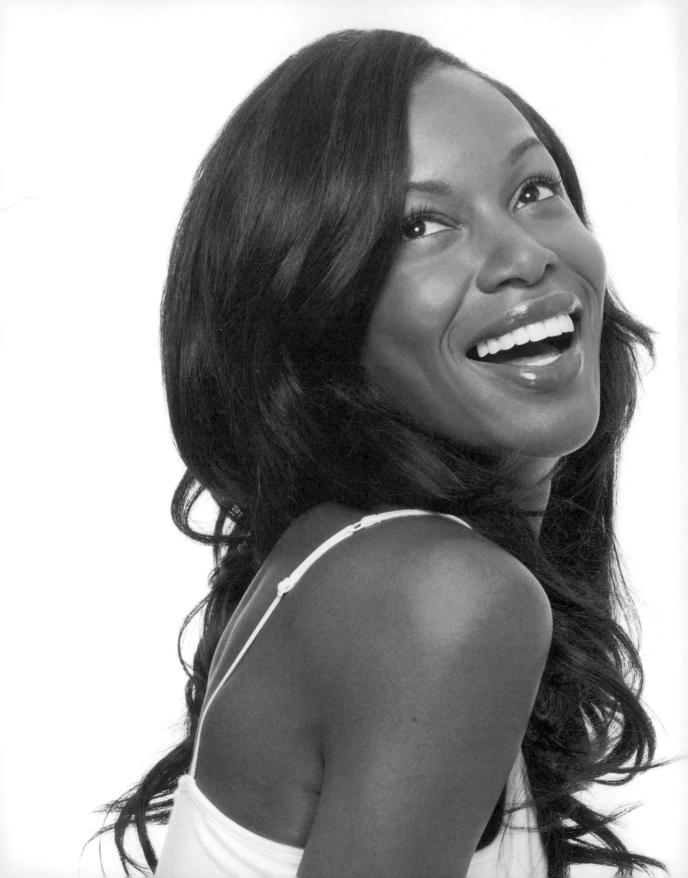

chapter 1

Face

Acne, Breakouts, Pimples, + Zits

Thought breakouts would remain in your past along with memories of middle school dances and teenage love? Unless you're one of the extraordinarily fortunate few for whom a breakout is more likely to mean a dance move than a zit (in which case you can just flip to the next chapter because clearly you don't need me here), blemishes happen to the best of us. Heck, the entire Proactiv marketing platform is predicated on famous celebrities with pimples!

Whether it's one pimple or one hundred, there's nothing like a big ole blemish to suddenly open the flood gates to the depths of insecurity. You're sure it's all anyone sees, all they are thinking about, and that your beauty is defined by it. Even the barely-there, brilliantly concealed pimple can wreak havoc on your self-esteem. Or at least mine, anyway!

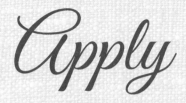

Apply

DIY Beauty Cures for Acne, Breakouts, Pimples, + Zits

If you're anything like me circa 2000, before I learned all I now know about using food for beauty, a pimple elicits an immediate fight-or-flight response. Assuming you can't hibernate for the next three to seven days until your blemish heals itself, you put on a suit of armor and pull out the big-guns: salicylic acid, benzoyl peroxide, sulfur, and retinols. You dive into your acne-annihilating arsenal, wage war on your skin, and likely come out on the other side pimpleless but with skin that more closely resembles the Sahara than your usually hydrated, supple, and smooth complexion. It's like dropping a nuclear bomb to kill an ant. Sure, it kills the ant, but at what expense?

Here's the deal: when you over-treat a blemish, you not only create a layer (or two!) of dry, dead skin that's ready, willing, and able to clog more pores at a moment's notice, but also inadvertently signal your skin to produce more oil to overcompensate your drying efforts, making you doubly prone to further breakouts!

So next time you notice a pimple (or a whole face full of them), step away from the medicine cabinet, meet me in the kitchen, and whip up these food-based pimple-purging recipes to treat breakouts naturally. Plus, you'll find a recipe from *Sports Illustrated* swimsuit model and actress Brooklyn Decker—a woman who not only has access to all the latest and greatest beauty products on the market, but whose career is dependent on her beauty.

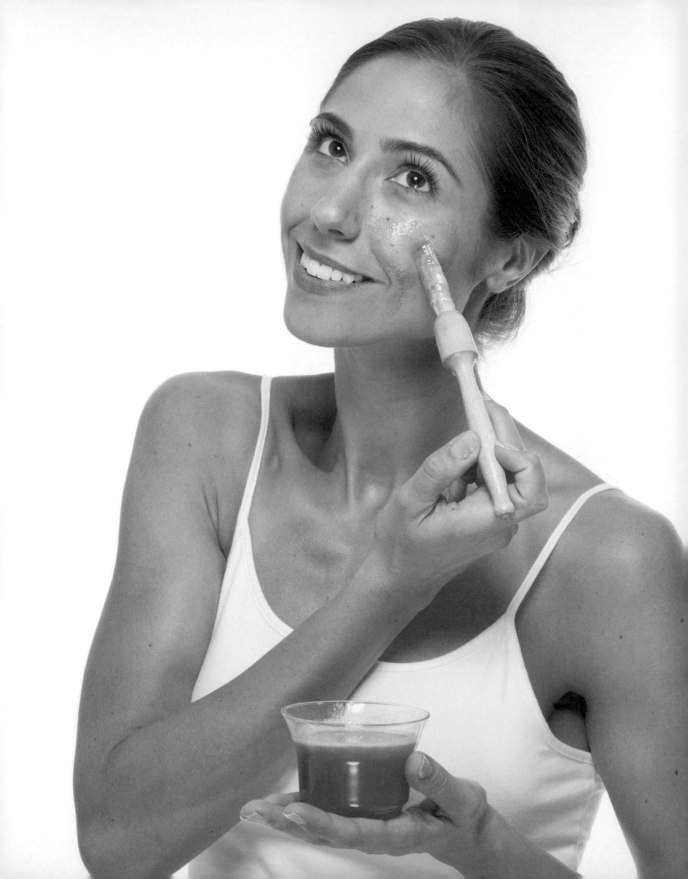

Hydrating + Blemish-Fighting Facial Mask

Dry, combination skin

If you have dry skin that's prone to breakouts, treating a pimple with traditional store-bought remedies can transport your face to desert-like conditions faster than an airplane ever could. Fortunately, drying out a pimple isn't the only way to send it packing. With antibacterial and hydrating honey, pore-tightening egg white, and exfoliating egg yolks, this facial mask will ensure your skin stays moisturized and supple while kicking breakouts to the curb. Egg yolks, with their fat, cholesterol, and retinols, are also great for helping to reduce the appearance of acne scars, making this ideal for post-pimple skin, too.

1 egg

1 tablespoon raw honey

Whisk the egg to fully combine the yolk and the white before stirring in the honey.

Use a pastry brush to apply a thin layer of the mixture to your face, neck, and décolleté, avoiding your eye area.

Let dry for 20 minutes to tighten pores, tone the skin, and kill bacteria, without drying your skin out.

Rinse with warm water and pat dry.

Note: Raw honey, available in any health food store, is creamy in consistency and considerably less sticky than regular honey, making it ideal for homemade beauty recipes—and well worth buying if you don't already own it.

"If you get a pimple, suffocate it! Just take a Band-Aid, rip off the two sticky ends, and then layer them in a cross on top of the blemish and wear it until morning. Ice helps too."

—Byrdie Bell, actress and model

Tropical Fruit Peel

From Mickey Williams, beauty expert

All skin types

Mickey Williams knows the benefits of layering on sunscreen while surfing in Costa Rica each year. But in much the same way sunscreen blocks the sun, it also blocks your pores. She says, "I basically layer and layer sunscreen until my skin freaks out and turns into a congested, salted hide." Instead of packing pricey masks or booking a facial at the hotel spa, Mickey hits the fridge for pineapple and papaya. "The natural enzymes are as powerful as a gentle peel or mask to break down the surface layer. If away for one week, I will usually apply the fruity love potion twice. It's super gentle and great for even sensitive skin." As an added bonus, it tastes great, so feel free to whip up extra and have it double as breakfast, too!

3 tablespoons puréed papaya
2 tablespoons puréed pineapple
1 tablespoon raw honey or plain yogurt

Stir all ingredients together until well combined.

Apply a thick layer to your skin, avoiding your eye area. Leave it on your skin for 10 minutes before rinsing with warm water.

Quick Tip

• Yogurt contains lactic acid, the same ingredient used in blemish-busting chemical peels! Next time you need a quick pimple-fighting fix, apply a thin layer of full-fat yogurt to the area for 10 minutes to calm and unclog.

Calming + Clearing Milk Mask

From Brooklyn Decker, model and actress

All skin types

Brooklyn Decker learned this homemade facial recipe from her favorite makeup artist in her hometown in North Carolina—and still relies on it to clear up a clogged complexion. "The sugar exfoliates my skin really well and the milk always calms my skin and gets rid of any redness," says Brooklyn. And, if it's good enough for this stunner, it's good enough for the rest of us, right?

½ cup white sugar
¼ cup whole milk

Quickly mix the sugar into the milk to form a thick paste, without allowing the sugar to dissolve.

Immediately apply a thick layer to your face, avoiding your eye area.

Let dry, about 15 minutes, before rinsing off with warm water and patting dry.

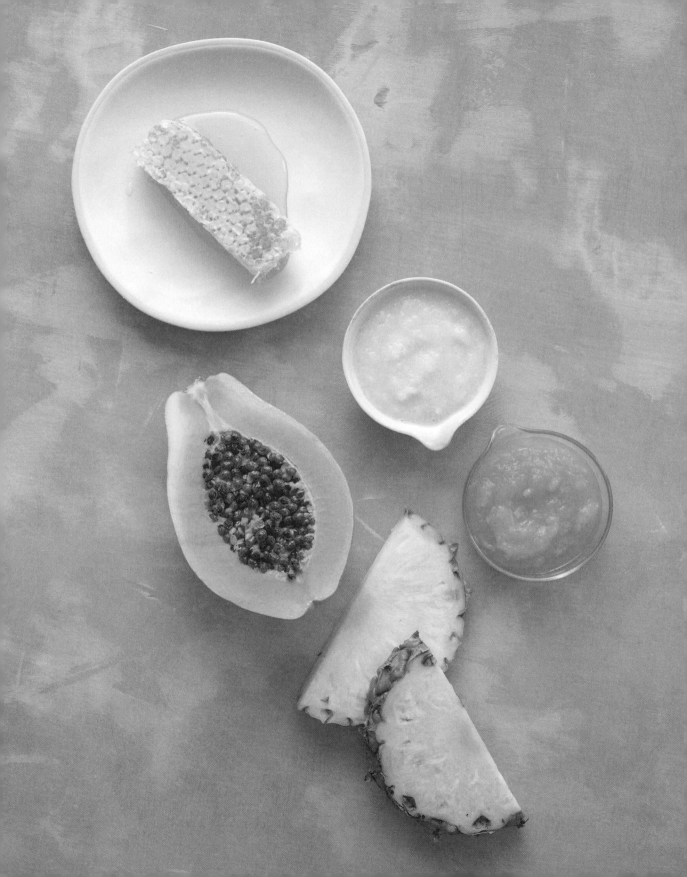

Anti-Acne Apple Astringent

Combination, oily skin

The high acidity of apple cider vinegar makes it an inhospitable environment for blemish-causing bacteria growth (which is also why so many holistic health practitioners advocate adding it to your diet, too!). Mixed with rosemary, a powerful astringent with anti-fungal properties, and mint, which helps to reduce redness and inflammation, this toner will not only help to keep skin clear from future breakouts but also will help to reduce the appearance and duration of any existing blemishes, too.

½ cup water

2 sprigs rosemary, chopped

2 tablespoons chopped mint leaves

½ cup apple cider vinegar

Bring water to a boil before adding the rosemary and the mint and reducing to a simmer for 10 minutes, uncovered.

Let cool to room temperature and strain before adding the vinegar.

Transfer to a spray bottle and store in the fridge. Shake well and spritz on clean skin before bed. Follow with nighttime moisturizer, if desired.

Quick Tips

• The inside of the peel of a banana is loaded with anti-inflammatory properties that can help reduce the redness and inflammation of a pimple. Peel off a piece of banana peel and turn it inside out so the white, fleshy part is exposed. Rub the peel over inflamed skin, leaving a thin coating of residue. Let the residue dry completely before using a warm washcloth to remove.

• Dissolve salt in warm water and apply it to any pimples with a cotton swab to dry out excess oils.

• Apple cider vinegar's high acidity makes it a bacteria-fighting blemish-buster. Just saturate a cotton ball and spot treat a pimple like actress Jen Lilley, who says, "Everyone should invest in apple cider vinegar. It's the best skin toner money can buy, and it's not even expensive!"

Eat

Food Cures for Acne, Breakouts, Pimples, + Zits

Chocolate and french fries may be the pimple-causing foods urban legends are made of, but, thankfully, they're just that: urban legends. While little scientific support exists for the idea of "pimple-causing foods," the fact is since your skin is your body's largest organ (yup, it's worth repeating!) and although there aren't any foods that "cause" breakouts, per se, there are certainly foods you can eat to help prevent breakouts from the inside out by supporting healthy, inflammation-free skin uninhibited by clogged pores.

Pores that are opened, clear, and oxygenated are inhabitable for pimple-causing bacteria. Unfortunately, for a lot of us, our skin doesn't turn over (beauty-insider speak for "exfoliate itself") as quickly as necessary to keep our pores clear. Think of it this way: Every day, we produce new skin cells and slough off old ones. Clogged pores occur when new cells appear but the old ones are still hanging on for dear life. One solution is to manually exfoliate them away with APPLY recipes, but another solution is to eat a diet rich in vitamin A, which helps your body to exfoliate from the inside out. Also important for an anti-acne diet are anti-inflammatory foods, which help to ensure that even when a pore does get clogged, it doesn't look like Jackson Pollock took red paint to your face.

Orange Sunshine Soup

Vegetarian, vegan, dairy-free, gluten-free

With vitamin A-rich carrots and yams, vitamin C-rich orange, and anti-inflammatory garlic and ginger, this creamy (but dairy-free) root vegetable soup supports healthy skin cell turnover from the inside out while also reducing redness and inflammation in acne-prone skin. Top with vitamin E-rich sunflower seeds to promote faster healing of existing blemishes from within and your skin will go from red to radiant in no time.

Serves 4

1 cup raw cashews

7 medium carrots, chopped

1 large garnet yam, peeled and cubed

2 tablespoons olive oil

3 cloves garlic, diced

½ white onion, chopped

1 large orange, peeled

2 cups low-sodium vegetable broth

2 tablespoons finely chopped ginger

½ teaspoon ground black pepper

4 tablespoons raw sunflower seeds

Soak the cashews in water and let sit for 30 minutes. Meanwhile, boil the carrots and the yam in water until soft, about 20 minutes.

In a separate pan, sauté the garlic and the onion in the oil, over medium heat, until slightly browned, about 5 to 7 minutes.

Drain the carrots, yam, and cashews and transfer to a food processor. Add the garlic, onions, orange, vegetable broth, ginger, and pepper and purée until smooth. (If your blender or food processor isn't large enough to process all of the ingredients, puree them separately and then stir them together in a large bowl.)

In a dry skillet, toast the sunflower seeds until fragrant and slightly golden.

Divide the soup into 4 bowls and top each with 1 tablespoon of the toasted sunflower seeds.

"Cut out simple carbs and increase your protein intake. Simple carbohydrates are metabolized as sugar and can radically affect hormonal balance, while whole grains and lean proteins can prevent breakouts."

—Suki Kramer, founder and president of suki skincare

Asian Cabbage Slaw

Vegetarian, vegan, dairy-free, gluten-free

Cabbage may not seem like a nutrient-packed powerhouse, but with indole-3-carbinol, a powerful antioxidant that supports detoxification in the liver, its cleansing benefits aren't to be overlooked. It's pretty much the reason for the Cabbage Soup Diet. And while I most definitely don't advocate a soup-based diet plan, adding this salad to your diet is a step in the right direction on the way to acne-free skin! Here's why: In helping to detoxify your liver, cabbage can help flush out the toxicities in your body, rather than letting them build up in your bloodstream, ultimately wreaking havoc on your skin. Combined with healthy fats (like those found in almonds and sesame seeds) to keep skin hydrated, this salad is a deliciously crunchy way to a clear complexion.

Serves 2 to 4

4 tablespoons apple
   cider vinegar
6 tablespoons toasted
   sesame oil
6 tablespoons honey
½ teaspoon salt
½ head red or green
   cabbage, shredded
2 scallions, chopped
¾ cup almond slivers
2 tablespoons sesame
   seeds
1 cup extra firm tofu
   (optional)

In a small bowl, whisk together the vinegar, toasted sesame oil, honey, and salt. (If the honey is difficult to stir, warm it by running the bottle under hot water to soften.)

Toss the chopped cabbage and scallions with the dressing. Cover and refrigerate for 1 to 2 hours.

Toast almond slivers in a dry skillet until fragrant and slightly browned.

Repeat with sesame seeds. (The almonds and sesame seeds will toast at different rates, so do them separately and watch each carefully.)

Toss the almonds and sesame seeds into the salad immediately prior to serving.

Top with tofu, if desired.

Note: If your acne is hormonally driven (often appearing around that time of the month and on your chin), skip the tofu in this recipe, as it may exacerbate hormonal blemishes.

Quick Tip

- Take a shot . . . of chlorophyll! As the building block of plants, it is loaded with anti-inflammatory and detoxifying properties, which is why celebrity facialist Cecilia Wong (who counts Lauryn Hill as a client) suggests adding a shot of this green, tasteless liquid to a morning glass of water for more beautiful skin from the inside out.

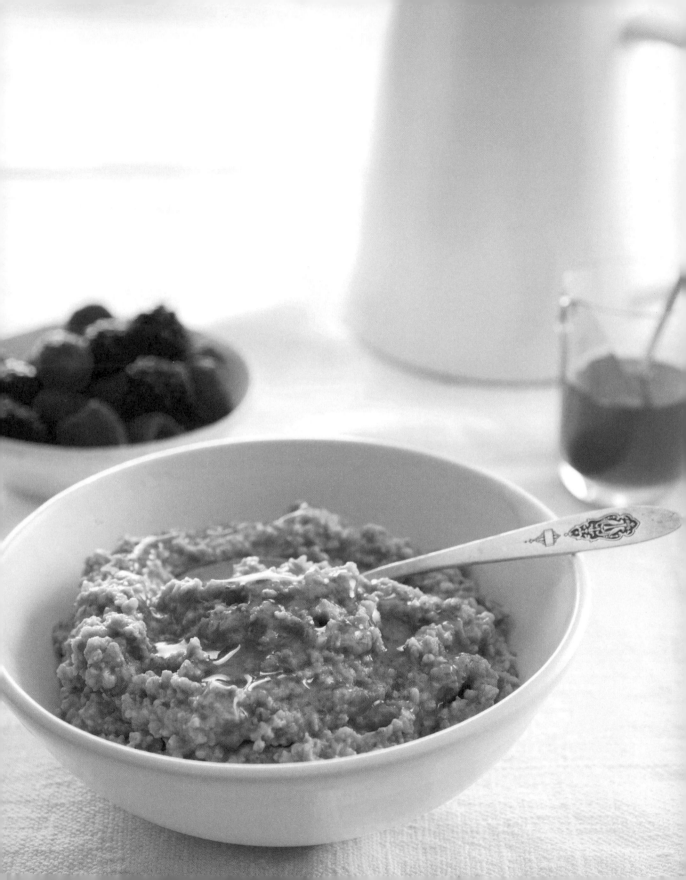

Raw Oatmeal

From Juice Press, New York City
Vegetarian, vegan, dairy-free

One cup of oats contains over sixteen grams of fiber, which not only helps keep you full for longer, but also helps to keep blood glucose and insulin levels stable, which, when high, can increase acne inflammation, particularly if you suffer with cystic acne. It's why in cultures with a diet free from insulin-spiking processed foods, acne is virtually nonexistent. To keep blood sugar steady (and cystic acne at bay)—deliciously, no less!—start your day off with a blood-sugar stabilizing breakfast like this raw oatmeal from Juice Press, one of my favorite raw food and juice places in New York City.

Serves 2

1 cup steel cut oats, soaked

½ cup cashews, soaked

12 medjool dates, pitted

¼ teaspoon vanilla extract

2 tablespoons extra-virgin cold-pressed coconut oil, liquefied

¼ teaspoon sea salt

Fresh berries (optional)

In separate bowls, soak the oats and the cashews overnight in enough filtered water to cover each.

Strain the cashews before placing them in a high-powered blender with the dates, vanilla extract, coconut oil, and salt. Add ¾ cup water. Blend until creamy, about 30 seconds.

Strain the soaked oats and put into a mixing bowl. Add the blended cashew milk to the oats and stir until well combined.

Cover and refrigerate for 20 minutes before serving.

Top with fresh berries, if desired.

Quick Tips

• Add lemon to your water to increase its detoxifying and alkalinizing properties to help flush out acne-causing toxins. Your skin will thank you.

• Extra-virgin cold-pressed coconut oil is one of the healthiest and most beauty-boosting cooking oils because of its unique acids and fats that make it not only beautify from the inside out, but also when applied topically. Plus, it's been shown to help burn belly fat!

Fine Lines + Wrinkles

For some people, it's a milestone birthday, for me I was going off to college when I first freaked out over my (inevitably) aging skin. Yes, I was eighteen. Yes, I was kinda crazy. Yes, I was destined to be a beauty editor. Whether you notice your first fine lines at fourteen or forty, the fact is that we're all destined to age. Just because we grow older, though, doesn't mean we have to look it (or—even scarier!—go under the knife).

Want to know the secret to looking younger? Or how one woman can look ten years older than another woman of the same age? It's not just genetics and it's not just sun exposure, although both most definitely play a role. A lot of it has to do with how you protect your skin from the inside out and outside in, both of which you can do with food found in your kitchen.

Apply

DIY Beauty Cures for Fine Lines + Wrinkles

Before you go out and spend a boat-load of cash on all the latest anti-aging products on the market (and yes, there are loads of them on which you could spend your hard-earned money), head to your kitchen instead. Not only are these homemade beauty remedies more cost-effective than the slew of store-bought anti-aging skincare products on the market vying for your money, many of them are even more effective than those you can buy at the store.

Here's why: a lot of the antioxidants that most effectively protect our skin from the aging effects of free radicals, stress, and life in general, are found in their most pure form in nature, and are most effective when fresh. And even store-bought skincare products that contain these fresh, active ingredients—with shelf lives upward of six months—are anything but fresh. It's like the difference between strawberries and strawberry jam. Sure, there is the convenience factor of buying a cream (or jam) that can sit in your home for months on end—and on the shelf at the store even longer—but as with your diet, when it comes to your skin care, fresh is often better. And, with such easy and affordable anti-aging recipes, why not fight the signs of aging naturally?

Age-Reversing Wine Mask

All skin types

In much the same way that red wine is anti-aging from the inside out, the antioxidants in red wine (including resveratrol) make it a great anti-aging skincare treatment when applied topically. Mixed with egg whites to tighten fine lines and retinol-rich egg yolks, this mask takes happy hour to a whole new level.

1 egg
1 egg yolk
3 tablespoons red wine

Whisk all ingredients together until well combined.

Use a pastry brush to apply a thin layer to your face, neck, and décolleté, avoiding your eye area.

Let dry before washing off with warm water and a washcloth.

Strawberry + Champagne Serum

Not for sensitive skin

Bet you didn't know that the grape seed extract in champagne packs more vitamin C and E than most anti-aging toners on the market, huh? Well, now you do! Next time you pop open a bottle of bubbly, set an ounce aside to make a potent anti-aging toner. Strawberries not only instantly brighten your complexion with their fruit acids but also simultaneously protect skin from further free radical damage with their antioxidant vitamin C, so this toner will reduce the appearance of fine lines and wrinkles while also helping to prevent further aging.

2 large strawberries, destemmed
1 ounce champagne

Muddle strawberries in a glass before mixing with champagne.

Use a cotton pad to apply a thin layer to your clean skin, avoiding your eye area, before bed.

In the morning, cleanse and moisturize as usual.

Quick Tips

• Actress Ginnifer Goodwin washes her face with organic extra-virgin cold-pressed coconut oil, which, she says, "is something everybody can do." It's antibacterial and hydrating, making it ideal for all skin types—and it removes even the most stubborn makeup!

• Apply all your anti-aging products (and DIY remedies!) to the backs of your hands, too—they're one of the first places to show signs of aging and are far too often neglected.

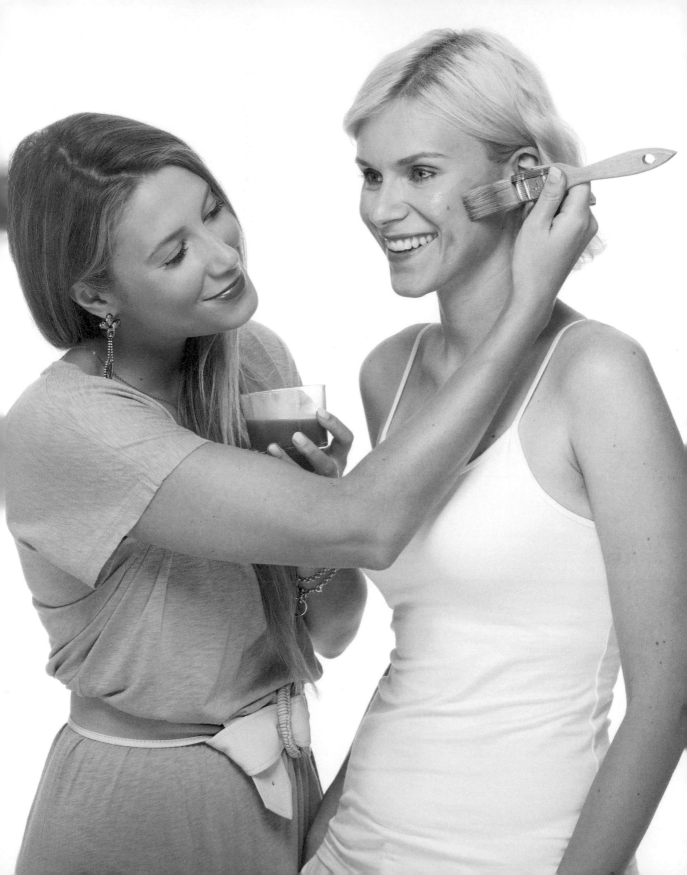

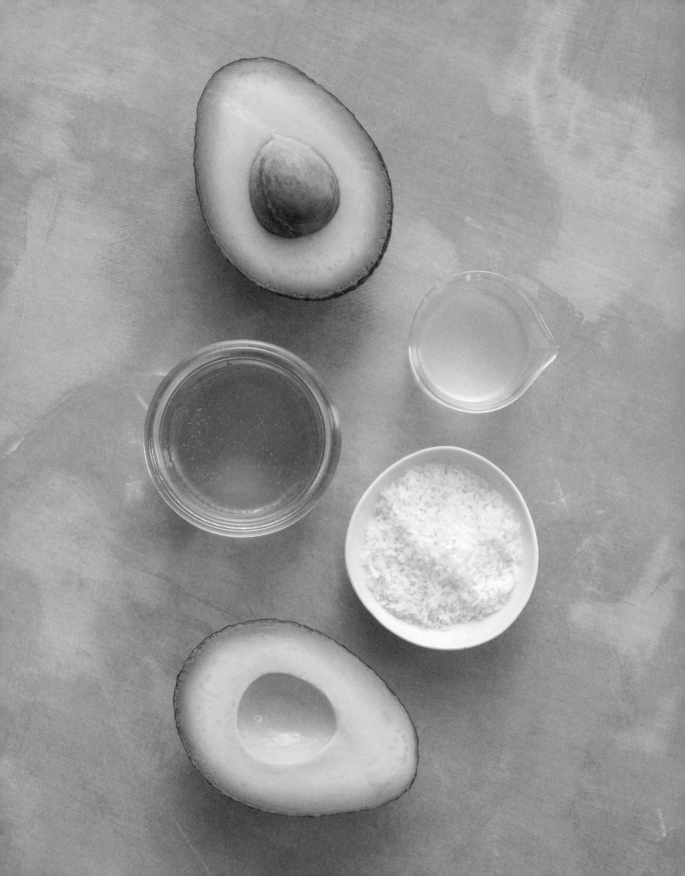

Piña Colada Polish

All skin types

Next time your skin is looking worn out and in need of a vacation, give it the skincare equivalent of a tropical getaway. With plumping omega-3 fatty acid from avocado, brightening pineapple fruit acids, hydrating honey, and exfoliating coconut shreds, this tropical exfoliating scrub will reveal brighter, more supple, younger-looking skin—stat!

2 tablespoons avocado

1 teaspoon fresh pineapple juice

1 teaspoon raw honey

2 tablespoons unsweetened coconut, shredded

Use a fork to mash the avocado until smooth. Stir in pineapple juice, honey, and coconut shreds.

Apply a thin layer to your skin, avoiding your eye area.

Let it sit for 10 minutes before using gentle, circular motions to exfoliate dead skin cells.

Rinse with warm water and pat dry.

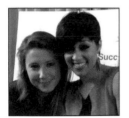

Quick Tip

- Actress Tia Mowry freezes brewed green tea in an ice cube tray and rubs it on her face to look younger. Just rub it on your face in the morning before applying moisturizer. The green tea's antioxidants are great for anti-aging, and the coldness decreases puffiness and tightens your pores.

"I learned this trick from an aesthetician at the Caudalie Vinothérapie Spa in New York a few years ago: Cut a chilled (almost frozen) seedless red or green grape in half, then slide the flat side over your face. Start between your brows then move out toward your temples. Go up your forehead, then down your nose and over your cheeks. Grapes are a powerful natural antioxidant which is great for fighting free radicals. Plus, the cooling sensation feels amazing on a hot summer day."

—Andrea Lavinthal, style director for People.com

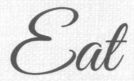

Eat

Food Cures for
Fine Lines + Wrinkles

Forget about the Fountain of Youth. It's the food of youth that you need to know about. With an anti-aging diet loaded with foods high in antioxidants, including flavonoids, carotenoids, vitamins, and minerals that work to neutralize free radicals (those pesky environmental factors that lead to premature aging), you really can eat your way to younger-looking skin.

The biggest aging offender: sun damage. Thankfully, though, with antioxidant-rich foods you can give yourself a hefty dose of SPF from the inside out. That's not to say you don't need SPF—if, as a beauty expert I can give you just one piece of advice it is this: Always. Wear. SPF. But by eating for beauty, you can tap into the real fountain of youth: food. And you don't need to compromise flavor in the process.

Seared Tuna with Mushroom + Scallion "Fried" Brown Rice

**From Michael Ferraro, executive chef/partner
at Delicatessen, New York City and *Iron Chef America* challenger**

Dairy-free, nut-free

Salmon may get all the attention when it comes to anti-aging fish, but tuna's not to be overlooked. Rich in selenium, a trace mineral shown to help prevent cellular damage, both tuna and brown rice help to ward off the environmental causes of aging, while simultaneously promoting the production of elastin, a protein in your connective tissue that keeps your skin unlined and wrinkle-free.

Serves 2

4 ounces tuna, sushi grade

1 tablespoon extra-virgin olive oil, divided

Salt and pepper, to taste

1 tablespoon sesame seeds

¼ cup minute brown rice

¼ cup vegetable stock

¼ cup shiitake mushrooms

1 clove garlic

½ teaspoon finely chopped ginger

1 tablespoon soy sauce

½ teaspoon white sugar

½ teaspoon wasabi paste

1 scallion stalk, thinly sliced

Slice the tuna into 3 thick pieces, keeping them together.

Add ½ teaspoon oil to a non-stick pan under medium-high heat.

Season tuna with salt and pepper and crust with sesame seeds. Place the tuna in the pan and cook for 1 minute. Rotate and cook four sides for 1 minute each.

Cook the rice in the vegetable stock according to the rice instructions.

In the non-stick pan, add the remaining oil, mushroom, garlic, and ginger and sauté over high heat for 2 minutes. Add the cooked rice and combine. Add in the soy sauce, sugar, and wasabi paste and combine evenly.

Press the rice into bottom of the pan, allowing the rice to slightly crisp, about 2 minutes.

Remove the rice and fold in the scallions.

Serve the rice with the tuna, fanned out, on top.

Quick Tip

• If you usually sip on soda or processed fruit drinks, try guava juice instead—the tropical fruit is packed with vitamin C, which boosts collagen production, for younger-looking skin.

Chilled Thai Almond Butter Noodles

Vegetarian, vegan, dairy-free

If you love pasta or Asian food—and especially if you love both—this is for you! Made from buckwheat, soba noodles contain monounsaturated fatty acids, which keep skin supple, as well as rutin, a flavonoid that may help improve skin's elasticity. Paired with a vitamin C-rich bell pepper, vitamin A-packed carrot, and vitamin E-filled almond butter, these cold and spicy noodles are like a time machine in a bowl (well, almost).

Serves 4 to 6

⅔ cup almond butter

3 tablespoons green
  curry paste

1 cup light coconut milk

1 tablespoon soy sauce

1 Thai chili pepper, diced
  (optional)

½ pound soba noodles

1 red bell pepper, julienned

1 large carrot, julienned

½ cup basil, chopped,
  divided

1 lime, to garnish

In a small saucepan, over low heat, warm the almond butter, curry paste, coconut milk, and soy sauce, stirring until well combined. Add the diced Thai chili pepper, if desired, for more heat.

Cook the soba noodles according to package instructions. When done, drain and plunge in cold water to cool.

Toss the noodles with half of the sauce to coat. Refrigerate both the noodles and the remaining sauce to chill (at least 2 hours). When chilled, toss the noodles with the remaining sauce, red pepper, carrot, and ¼ cup basil.

Top with the remaining basil and lime wedges to serve.

Quick Tip

• Snack on Brazil nuts. They're loaded with selenium, a mineral that helps to repair damaged cells and slow down the skin's aging process.

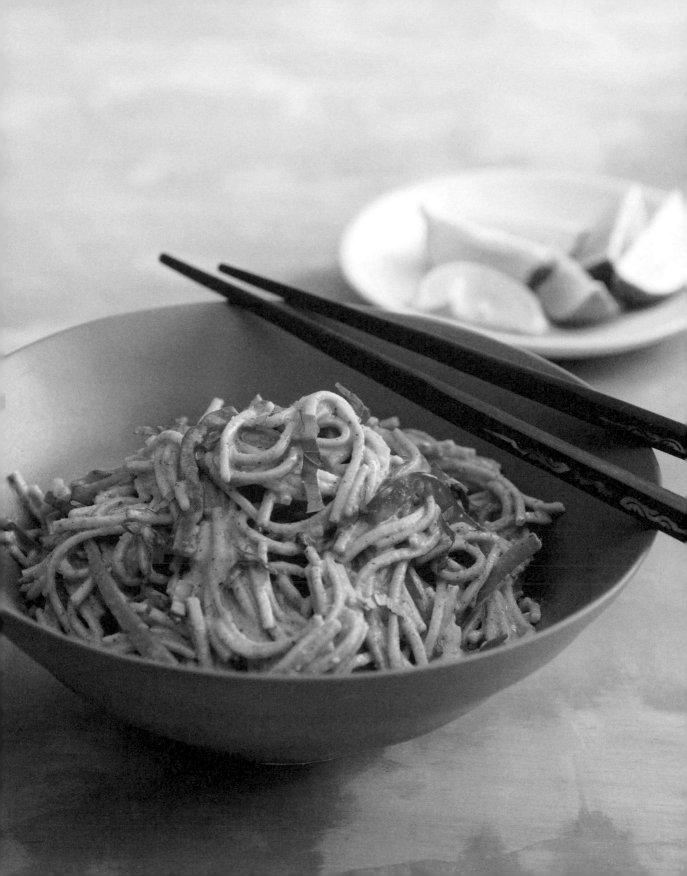

Almond Butter + Strawberries

Vegetarian, vegan, dairy-free, gluten-free

Like peanut butter and jelly, this is a crowd favorite! Sure to satisfy your inner child (even if your skin is far from child-like), the strawberries in this antioxidant-crammed snack help protect your skin from further aging with their vitamin C, while the vitamin E in the almond butter helps to smooth existing fine lines and wrinkles from the inside out. I like making my own raw almond butter to ensure it's organic, raw, and sugar- and salt-free. If you buy your own, just be sure it's raw and organic with almonds as the only ingredient.

Serves 2 to 4

½ cup raw almonds

1 tablespoon raw honey

1 pint strawberries, destemmed

Almond oil, if needed

Puree almonds and honey in a high-powered blender until a thick nut butter forms, about 5 minutes. Add almond oil, if needed, to thin the consistency.

Meanwhile, wash and destem the strawberries before slicing them in half.

Top each strawberry half with a dollop of homemade almond butter and serve immediately.

Quick Tip

• Dehydrating fruit can cause some nutrients to become more concentrated, making dried fruit an antioxidant power-house. Just steer clear of sweetened varieties.

Sea Greens Salad

Lee Gross, consulting chef at M Café, Los Angeles
Vegetarian, vegan, dairy-free, gluten-free, nut-free

Sea vegetables may not be a regular part of your diet, but they should be! In fact, they are packed with such copious beauty benefits that deciding which chapter to put this recipe in was a challenge, because it could go in almost any one!

An ancient beauty secret of Japanese women who consume them regularly, sea vegetables are extraordinarily nutrient-rich—with some varieties having more protein, iron, and B vitamins than eggs, beef, and oysters, respectively. All of these elements work together to regenerate, revitalize, protect, and oxygenate skin from the inside out. Bottom line: they're like beauty in a bite.

Serves 4 to 6

1 teaspoon grated or finely minced ginger

¼ teaspoon grated or finely minced garlic

3½ tablespoons rice vinegar

3 tablespoons shoyu (natural soy sauce) or tamari

1 teaspoon natural sweetener (brown rice syrup, agave, or maple syrup)

3 tablespoons toasted sesame oil

3 ounces mixed dry sea vegetables

1 small green apple, chopped

2 scallions, thinly sliced

1 large or 2 small radishes, thinly sliced

1 stalk celery, chopped

½ small head Napa cabbage, chopped

2 tablespoons cilantro, chopped

1 tablespoon sesame seeds, toasted

Whisk the ginger, garlic, vinegar, shoyu, sweetener, and sesame oil to combine.

Place the dry sea vegetables in a deep bowl and cover with lukewarm water. Let it sit for 10 minutes to reconstitute.

Drain well, and chop any large leaves into bite-size pieces.

Place the reconstituted sea vegetables, apple, scallions, radish, celery, cabbage, cilantro, and sesame seeds in a large bowl and mix well to combine. Add dressing, to taste. Mix well to coat all ingredients.

For a fresh, crunchy salad, serve immediately. Or, for a more flavorful, marinated salad, refrigerate for 30 minutes to 1 hour.

Note: Sea vegetables are available at any Asian market, or can be created by any combination of wakame, arame, hijiki, and kelp noodles.

Age Spots + Hyperpigmentation

If you were born before the Stay-Out-of-the-Sun memo most of us (or our parents) got circa 1985, you likely acquired quite a bit of sun damage before you were even old enough to actively rebel against seemingly silly rules, like wearing wrist guards when rollerblading. Emphasis on "seemingly." I learned my lesson the hard way that full-body armor should be in order when taking part in any activity that involves balancing on blades of any kind. (I still have a scar commemorating the cuts and scrapes I got when I thought it would be a blast to rollerblade down a big hill in fifth grade without any braking skills to speak of whatsoever). Here's hoping you similarly learned your lesson when it comes to the dangers of too much sun exposure.

As I'm sure you now (hopefully!) gear up appropriately for activities that pose risks easily assuaged by a bit of protective gear (helmets when biking, harnesses when rock climbing, condoms when having sex), you hopefully also gear up for daily life with a protective application of SPF. That doesn't mean that the effect of too many rebellious or merely absentminded days spent in the sun haven't already done their damage. You're apt to have sunspots or hyperpigmentation to show for it.

Unfortunately, the most common over-the-counter and prescription products for reducing the appearance of sun and age spots contain hydroquinone, a chemical that has actually been banned in cosmetics in Europe because of its potential cancer-causing properties. Yikes! Also common, and even more aggressive, are lasers and chemical peels that not only require a serious financial investment but also often require some serious downtime to recover. Fortunately, your kitchen may have just the solution you're looking for.

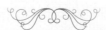

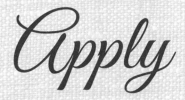

Apply

DIY Beauty Cures for Age Spots + Hyperpigmentation

Unless you want to call your brown spots "beauty marks" (more power to you if that's your game plan!), the key to reducing the appearance of age spots or other forms of hyperpigmentation is to speed up cell turnover and encourage your skin to heal itself and slough off those darkened (i.e. damaged) skin cells. It's how chemical peels and lasers work, too: by speeding up your skin's natural exfoliating process. And while they usually get the job done (after you sacrifice your first born, or at the very least your rent money and multiple layers of skin), lasers and chemical peels often cause serious bruising and unsightly reptile-like peeling, respectively, leaving you out of commission for days or even weeks.

For a more wallet-, time-, and skin-friendly approach, encourage cell turnover naturally with ingredients in your kitchen. Sure, the results will reveal themselves a bit more slowly than a chemical peel, but without a week or more of recovery time I say it's well worth the wait.

Pumpkin Key Lime Brightener

All skin types

If you're a pumpkin or key lime pie fan, you're going to eat up this dark-spot-reversing scrub. Combining the vitamin A of the pumpkin, the citric acid of the lime, and the lauric acid of the coconut oil, this scrub works to break down damaged, darkened skin cells that the sugar can then manually exfoliate away. At the same time, the vitamin C and citric acids in the key lime juice help to brighten your skin to further reduce the appearance of dark spots.

2 tablespoons pumpkin, fresh and puréed or canned
1 key lime, juiced
1 tablespoon extra-virgin cold-pressed coconut oil
3 tablespoons white sugar

Combine all of the ingredients in a small bowl to form a thick paste.

Apply to darkened areas, avoiding your eye area. Let it sit for 10 minutes before gently scrubbing away.

Rinse remnants off with warm water.

Geisha's Secret Sake Serum

All skin types

With this topical hyperpigmentation remedy—based on an ancient geisha beauty secret—next time you spill a drink on yourself, it may not be so bad after all. Sake has an acid that, when applied topically, diminishes your body's ability to create the melanin responsible for sun spots. Mixed with orange and lemon juice, both high in ascorbic and citric acids, this sake toner will help fade sun and age spots while also cleansing, protecting, and brightening your skin. This APPLY recipe is more potent than any store-bought skin-care products that boast of sake as an ingredient since the active properties aren't stable enough to be included in store-bought skin care! So, say "sayonara" to those age spots once and for all.

1 ounce unfiltered sake
½ ounce freshly squeezed orange juice
½ ounce freshly squeezed lemon juice

In a small bowl, combine all of the ingredients.

With a cotton pad, apply a thin layer to clean skin, avoiding your eye area.

For a deeper treatment, saturate cotton pads with the toner and lay on your skin for 10 minutes.

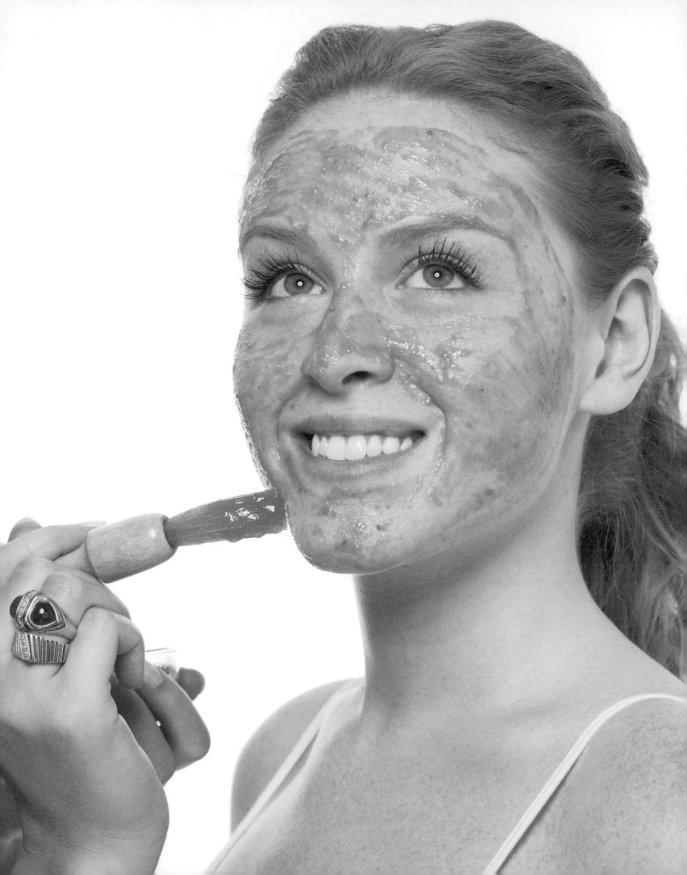

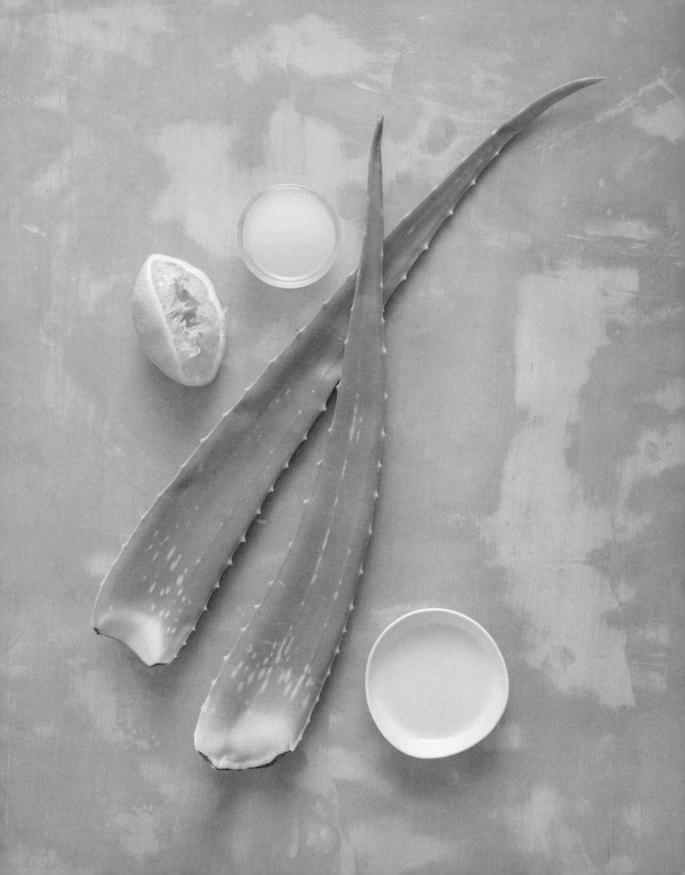

Skin-Lightening Spot Treatment

All skin types

With soy milk to counter the melanin in your skin responsible for the darkening, lemon to help exfoliate away the outer most—and darkest—layer of your skin, and aloe to speed up your own body's healing processes, when used daily this spot treatment will help to gradually fade dark spots. Just remember: your sun spots didn't appear overnight, and neither will they disappear immediately. With regular application of this spot treatment, though, your dark spots will steadily fade until you never even knew they were there.

1 tablespoon soy milk

1 tablespoon lemon juice

1 tablespoon aloe vera juice (from the leaf or bottled)

Combine all of the ingredients in a small bowl. Use a cotton swab to spot treat age or sun spots twice a day.

Cover with SPF if going outside.

Quick Tips

• You know why celebs are always in hats and sunnies? Nope, it's not just to hide from the paparazzi—although that's surely a factor. It's because they know that sun damage is what leads to those unsightly dark spots. So, take note and invest in hats and sunglasses. You may feel like such a rock star you won't even want to take them off.

• In a rush? Apply lemon juice to a cotton swab and apply directly to hyperpigmented areas to break down darkened skin cells. The sooner you notice a sunspot, the sooner you should treat it. The younger they are, the better they respond to treatment.

"Of course, we all know the skincare benefits of regular, gentle exfoliation. I have a recipe that was born out of necessity while traveling. It worked so well that I decided to stick with it. Add one packet of white sugar (if you're traveling) or one tablespoon of sugar if you're home to about two tablespoons of a gentle cleanser. Mix and apply to skin in gentle, circular motions. After a few seconds, the sugar crystals begin to dissolve. The sugar-and-cleanser combo is a super gentle, cost-effective way to exfoliate skin. Rinse and follow with your favorite toner, serum, and face cream."

—Felicia Walker Benson of ThisThatBeauty.com

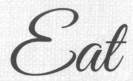

Eat

Food Cures for Age Spots + Hyperpigmentation

Sure, a healthy (not hefty) dose of vitamin D is important for your bones, mood, and even your complexion (assuming your idea of beauty doesn't involve a Johnny Depp in *Edward Scissorhands* level of pastiness), but in excess you run the risk of all the nasty effects of too much sun exposure including, but certainly not limited to, age spots and hyperpigmentation.

To protect your skin from sun damage from the inside out, antioxidants are key. But what about when the damage has been done? Are you destined to have a face freckled by age spots and a life spent trying to cover them up with makeup?

Of course not. By eating the right foods, you can help your body to heal and reverse sun damage from the inside out.

Nut Butter
Chicken Salad Wrap

Dairy-free, nut-free

Want to spice up your go-to chicken salad sandwich, with skin-brightening benefits to boot? Try this peanut buttery (but peanut-free) chicken salad sandwich instead! It includes sunflower seed butter, which boasts some of the highest concentrations of vitamin E, a vitamin necessary for healing everything from acne scars to sun spots from the inside out. The sandwich also has high-protein grilled chicken, important for cellular growth, and is served in a whole-wheat wrap, which is rich in skin-saving selenium. This unique take on your traditional chicken salad sandwich may just be your new go-to favorite—or at least your skin's new favorite!

Serves 2

2 teaspoons honey

2 tablespoons sunflower seed butter

2 tablespoons mayonnaise

8 ounces chicken, grilled and cubed

½ Fuji or gala apple, diced

1 stalk celery, diced

½ cup red grapes, halved

2 whole-wheat wraps

In a mixing bowl, combine the honey, sunflower seed butter, and mayonnaise, stirring until smooth. Add the chicken, apple, celery, and grapes.

Divide between the whole-wheat wraps, wrap, and serve immediately.

If you prefer to prepare this ahead of time, keep fruit separate until immediately prior to serving, to prevent the salad from getting watery.

Quick Tip

• Most of the age-spot reducing vitamins—namely vitamins A and E—are fat-soluble, meaning you need to eat them with at least a little bit of fat for them to do their age-spot-reducing work.

Pumpkin Pie Pancakes + Cranberry Maple Syrup

Vegetarian, nut-free

With beta-carotene-packed pumpkin, these pancakes take a favorite breakfast staple to a sun-spot reducing new level. Even better, the cranberries in the compote are jam-packed with antioxidants, so you'll be protected from new sun spots as well. Double up the batch and freeze half for an easy age-spot reducing breakfast even when you're in a hurry.

Serves 4 to 6

4 cups cranberries

⅓ cup maple syrup

1 can (15 ounces) pumpkin purée

1 ½ cups vanilla almond milk, unsweetened

2 eggs

½ cup extra-virgin olive oil

1 ½ tablespoons agave

1 teaspoon vanilla

1 ½ cups whole-wheat flour

3 ½ teaspoons baking powder

½ teaspoon cinnamon

¼ teaspoon nutmeg

¼ teaspoon salt

In a small sauce pan, over medium-high heat, combine the cranberries and the maple syrup. Bring to a boil before reducing to a simmer for 6 to 8 minutes, stirring occasionally.

In a large mixing bowl, whisk the pumpkin, almond milk, eggs, oil, agave, and vanilla until smooth. Stir in the flour, baking powder, cinnamon, nutmeg, and salt, whisking for about 2 minutes, longer for fluffier pancakes.

On a nonstick (or pre-greased) griddle on medium-high heat, spoon the batter onto the griddle for about 3 minutes. Flip approximately halfway through, or when the surface begins to bubble.

Top with cranberry compote and serve immediately.

Quick Tip
• Snack on berries to help prevent age spots. Their antioxidants are like an internal SPF!

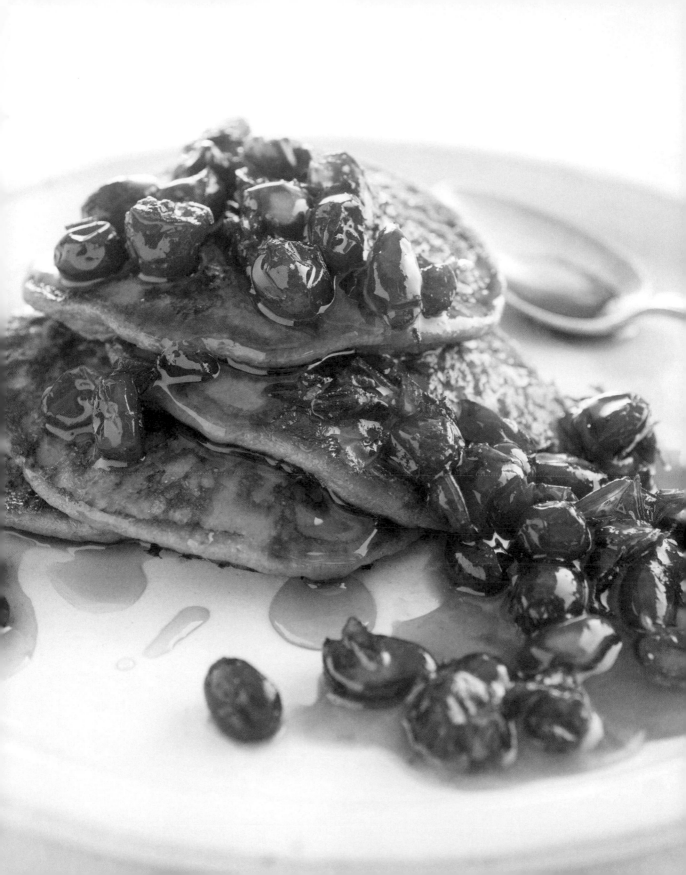

Green Papaya Salad

From David Gilbert, James Beard Award nominee and author of *Kitchen Vagabond*

Dairy-free, gluten-free

This dish is popular throughout South East Asia—mostly for its complexity of flavors, but I think you'll love it for the skin-brightening benefits, too! With papaya's skin-healing vitamins C and A, which reduce inflammation and encourage skin healing; tomatoes' skin-protecting lycopene, which acts like internal SPF; shrimp's rejuvenating protein; and cabbage's antioxidants, this Thai salad will help keep skin even-toned and age-spot free.

Serves 4

3 cloves garlic

2 to 3 Thai chilies

½ teaspoon dried small shrimp
(available at Asian markets)

1 tablespoon palm sugar

1 ½ cup green papaya,
julienned or cut lengthwise
on the mandolin

¼ cup Chinese long beans,
cut in 2-inch pieces

2 to 3 tablespoons fish sauce

1 tablespoon tamarind

1 tablespoon lime juice

4 cherry tomatoes, quartered

Crushed roasted peanuts,
to taste

Green cabbage, shredded,
to serve

Place the garlic, Thai chilies, dried shrimp, and palm sugar into a tall mortar and begin to break down with the pestle.

Add in the green papaya, long beans, fish sauce, tamarind, and lime juice and continue to bruise with the pestle, being sure to keep the salad crunchy, not limp from over-pounding.

Top with the cherry tomatoes. Adjust the seasonings as desired, for a balance of sweet, sour, and salty. Allow the mixture to sit for 8 to 10 minutes in the dressing.

Place in a bowl and garnish with the crushed peanuts. Serve with a side of green cabbage.

Sweet Potato Chips + Cumin Dip

Vegetarian, vegan, dairy-free, gluten-free, nut-free

Sweet potatoes, with their skin-rejuvenating vitamin A, are just the fuel you need on the road to eradicating those sun and age spots for good. Because vitamin A is fat-soluble though, it's important to eat it with a healthy fat, like avocado, in order to really reap the benefits. I like to think of this as the beauty-boosting and healthy alternative to potato chips and sour cream dip—and even yummier. Best of all for you chip lovers: you won't feel guilty after eating this version!

Serves 4 to 6

2 medium sweet potatoes, thinly sliced

1 tablespoon extra-virgin olive oil

1 ripe avocado

3 teaspoons lime juice

1 teaspoon cumin

¼ teaspoon salt

⅛ teaspoon black pepper

Preheat the oven to 350°F.

Toss the sweet potatoes with the oil and spread evenly on a baking sheet.

Bake for 1 hour, or until crispy, tossing half way through. If the chips on the edges bake more quickly, remove them and return the remainder to the oven to crisp.

In a small bowl, whisk the avocado with the lime juice, cumin, salt, and pepper. Refrigerate for 20 minutes to allow the flavors to meld before dipping.

Quick Tip
• Load up on dark orange vegetables (like carrots, sweet potatoes, and squash) to keep age spots away.

Redness + Rosacea

Does your skin get robustly rosy in the summer heat, piqued pink in the winter chill, and fiercely fired up whenever you exercise? Do you pick a pimple and stay red for ages? Or do you suffer with rosacea that leaves your skin ruddy all year long?

If a red face has you feeling green with envy for a creamy complexion, fret not.

Rather than attempting to nail the application of green-tinted makeup designed to counteract the redness in your skin, which, more often than not, leaves your skin looking Wicked Witch of the West-like—and dull to boot—let's get to the bottom of the issue and cure your facial redness rather than merely attempting to cover it up. Especially since even top makeup artists have a hard time perfectly applying green-tinted makeup!

Please note though, severe cases of rosacea, particularly those with pustules present, sometimes require prescription medications or laser treatments, although an anti-inflammatory diet and topical anti-inflammatory solutions will help.

The secret to treating facial redness, naturally, is in understanding its cause—and, no, I'm not talking about what predisposes you to redness (aka genetics) but rather what's actually happening within your skin that's leaving you red. Here's what you need to know: The redness you see when you look in the mirror is caused by the inflammation and dilation of the blood vessels immediately under your skin's surface. The key to eliminating your facial redness is both in constricting those dilated blood vessels and in reducing the redness-causing inflammation, the first of which we can treat topically and the latter we can tackle with an anti-redness diet.

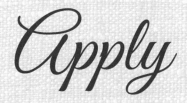

Apply

DIY Beauty Cures
for Redness + Rosacea

Inflammation is most often our body's way of healing itself. When you sprain your ankle and it immediately swells, it's your body's way of sending aid to the area. Unfortunately, like our minds, our bodies sometimes overreact, sending far more blood flow than is required. That sprained ankle of yours calls for ice because a mild sprain doesn't require as much increased blood flow as our bodies initially anticipate and, well, that swelling can end up doing more harm than good—at least to our ability to fit in our shoes. The same is true of our faces.

Like with a swollen ankle, when your face is inflamed with redness or puffiness, cooling the area can help, but these beauty recipes will ensure the benefits last far longer than an ice pack ever will, and prevent you from walking around with an ice-pack on your face all day.

Healing Herbal Tonic

All skin types

When it comes to constricting blood vessels, few ingredients are more effective than those rich in vitamin K. Essential for normal blood clotting, vitamin K helps promote blood vessel health from the inside out; and when applied topically, it helps to constrict blood vessels, especially those close to the skin's surface. With basil, sage, and thyme, all of which are abundant in vitamin K, this herbal toner will gently and effectively help to reduce facial blood flow and redness for a creamier complexion, naturally and without makeup.

¾ cup water
1 tablespoon dried basil
1 tablespoon dried sage
1 tablespoon dried thyme

Bring the water to a boil before adding the dried basil, sage, and thyme. Reduce heat and simmer, uncovered, until about half of the water has evaporated.

Remove from the heat and let cool to room temperature before straining.

Pour the toner into an empty bottle and refrigerate.

Apply to a cotton pad and gently apply to your face, after cleansing, both in the morning and at night.

For a more intensive redness-reducing treatment, saturate cotton pads with this herbal toner and let it sit on your face for 10 to 15 minutes.

Cooling Coffee Compresses

All skin types

Think coffee does wonders for your energy levels? Wait until you see what it can do for your skin! The caffeine in coffee is one of the best ways to constrict the dilated blood vessels bringing unwanted rosiness to your face (that's why so many creams for under-eye circles rely on this energy booster), making it an ideal remedy for alleviating facial redness. The key here, though, is in refrigerating the coffee to maximize its constricting properties.

1 cup caffeinated coffee

Brew 1 cup of strong, caffeinated coffee. (If your coffee machine allows, add twice the recommended amount of coffee for 1 cup of water to create an especially dark brew.)

Refrigerate overnight or until chilled.

Soak a washcloth or cotton pads in the brew and apply to your face for 10 to 15 minutes. Rinse clean with cool water.

Quick Tip
• Avoid washing your face with water that's too hot or too cold, since extreme temperatures force blood flow (aka redness) to your skin's surface.

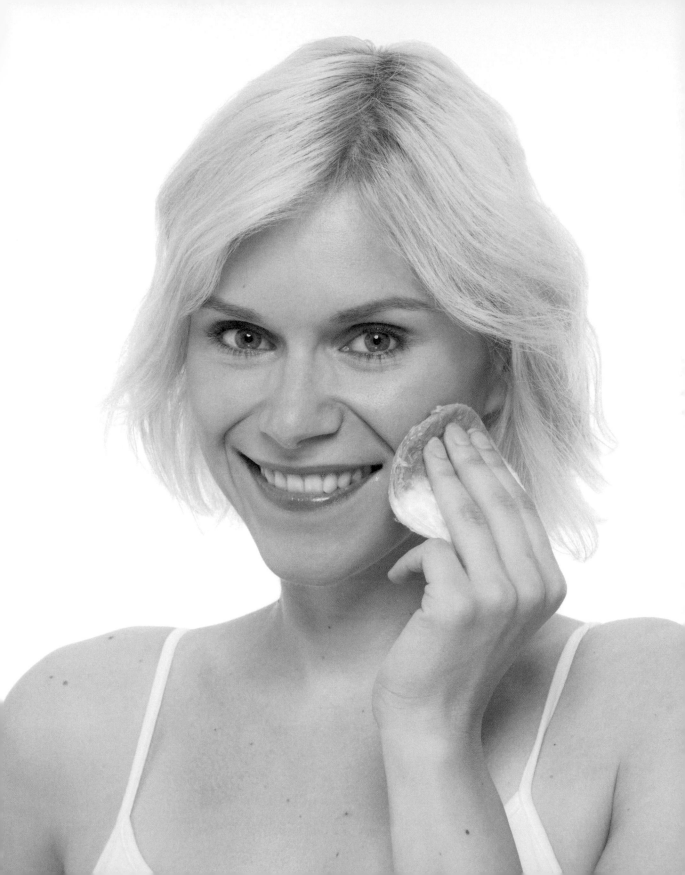

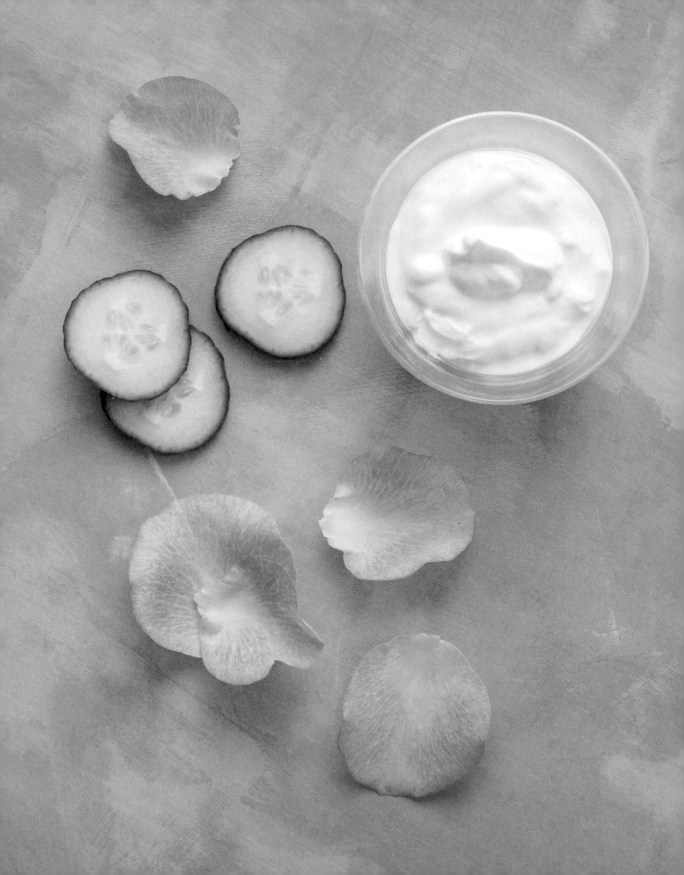

Cucumber + Rose Redness Remedy

From Jen Navaro, celebrity and editorial makeup artist

All skin types

While I've only had the pleasure of working with Jen Navaro once (on a Vidal Sassoon video shoot), I immediately connected with her all-natural approach to beauty. Quickly thereafter, I e-mailed her asking for a recipe for this book, knowing she'd have the inside scoop on some of the best tricks in the business.

As a former skincare pro turned makeup artist (whose work you likely saw in the last fashion magazine you read), Jen knows the importance of not merely concealing redness on photo shoots, but of actually getting to the root cause of it. Her go-to solution: this cucumber and rose mask. With rose water, a gentle, effective, and natural antiseptic that works wonders on rosacea/reactive skin types; cucumber to calm; and yogurt to reduce inflammation, this mask quickly and effectively cools, soothes, tones, and heals the skin.

½ **medium cucumber**

1 **rose in full bloom**

¼ **cup plain Greek yogurt**

Wash the wax off of the cucumber using a fruit and vegetable wash before roughly chopping.

Pluck the petals from the rose.

In a blender, puree the cucumber and rose petals until smooth.

Transfer to a mixing bowl and stir in the yogurt until well combined.

Place in the freezer for 15 minutes before applying liberally to clean skin (ideally after a warm shower, when pores are open).

Allow the mask to sit for 20 minutes before rinsing off with cool water. Follow with moisturizer.

"A cup of oatmeal mixed with a tablespoon of honey is a great face mask. Apply it for 15 minutes and rinse off. It helps reduce facial redness and keeps my skin looking youthful!"

—**Kristin Chenoweth, Tony Award-winning singer and actress**

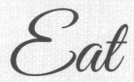

Eat

Food Cures
for Redness + Rosacea

While a propensity toward redness and rosacea is partly based on our genetic makeup, facial redness, no matter your family history, is not inevitable. Sure, some of us are more prone to a ruddy complexion or lingering redness after a workout, day in the sun, or time spent picking a blemish, but with an anti-inflammatory diet, you can help support your body's natural redness-reducing process for a less fiery complexion.

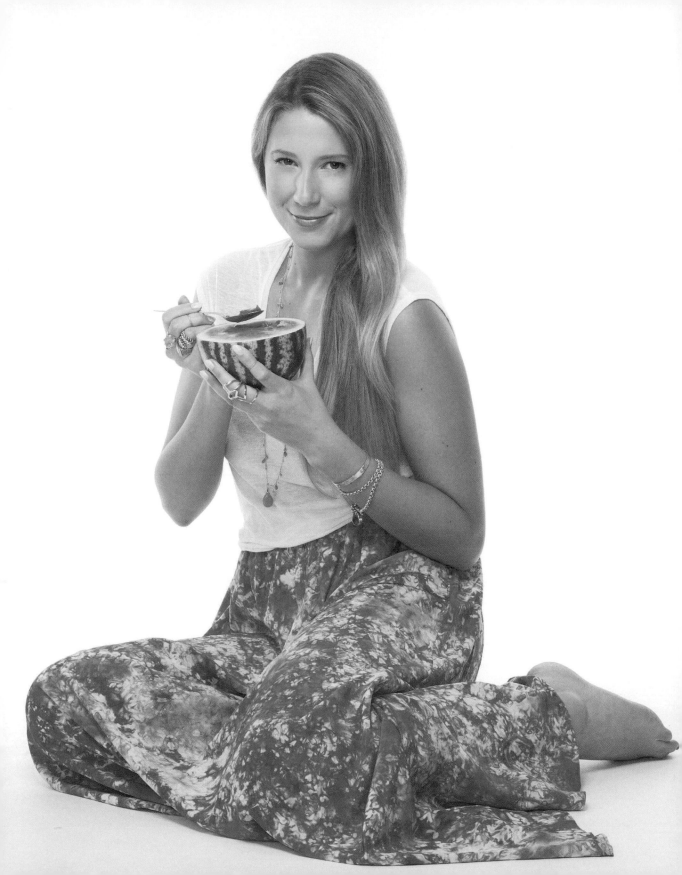

Mint + Ginger
Green Tea Lemonade

Vegetarian, vegan, dairy-free, gluten-free, nut-free

With cooling mint, anti-inflammatory ginger, antioxidant green tea, and detoxifying lemons, this drink will not only help sooth red, irritated skin from the inside out, but also make forgoing hot beverages (which can exacerbate facial redness) easier than ever.

Serves 4

4 cups water, divided

4 tea bags green tea

½ cup chopped fresh mint leaves, tightly packed

⅓ cup chopped fresh ginger

¼ cup agave

⅓ cup fresh lemon juice

Lemon slices, to garnish (optional)

Bring 2 cups of water to a boil before reducing to a simmer. Add the green tea bags, chopped mint, ginger, and agave and let steep 30 minutes.

Strain into a large pitcher, pressing on the solids to extract as much liquid as possible. Add the lemon juice and remaining water.

Refrigerate until chilled.

Serve over ice.

Quick Tips

• Avoid hot showers—or washing your face with hot water—both of which bring increased circulation to your skin.

• Rosemary contains ursolic and carnosic acids and plant compounds with powerful antioxidant and anti-inflammatory properties, so sprinkle it on vegetables and meats liberally!

Pan-Seared Sea Scallops +
Truffled Shiitake Rice

Dairy-free, gluten-free, nut-free

Asian mushrooms (like shiitake), brown rice, and heart-healthy oils are all anti-inflammatory. Combined with vitamin K-rich parsley to help with normal blood vessel functioning, you can rest assured this decadent rice dish will keep flushing at bay. Blushing, when compliments come a-flooding, however, is a whole other story!

Serves 2

2 cups cooked brown rice

¼ cup chopped flat-leaf parsley

4 tablespoons white truffle oil

½ teaspoon Himalayan sea salt

4 tablespoons extra-virgin olive oil, divided

1 leek, chopped

½ pound shiitake mushrooms, thickly sliced

½ cup dry white wine

4 large sea scallops

Parmesan cheese (optional)

Cook the brown rice according to package instructions. When the rice is cooked through, add the parsley, white truffle oil, and salt, stirring until combined. Set aside.

In a large skillet, heat 2 tablespoons olive oil over medium heat. Add the leeks and shiitake mushrooms and sauté until the mushrooms begin to soften, about 2 to 3 minutes. Add the wine and let simmer until liquid evaporates. Add to rice and set aside.

Wash and dry the scallops.

Place the remaining 2 tablespoons olive oil in skillet over high heat.

Add the washed and dried scallops, making sure they are not touching each other. Sear the scallops for 1 to 2 minutes on each side, until golden on the outside and still moist on the inside.

Serve over rice.

Top with shaved parmesan, if desired.

Quick Tips

• Stay away from spicy foods, which not only set your mouth on fire, but also dilate your blood vessels and can make your face look on fire!

• Keep all of your skincare products in the refrigerator for the cooling effect, as well as to increase their shelf life!

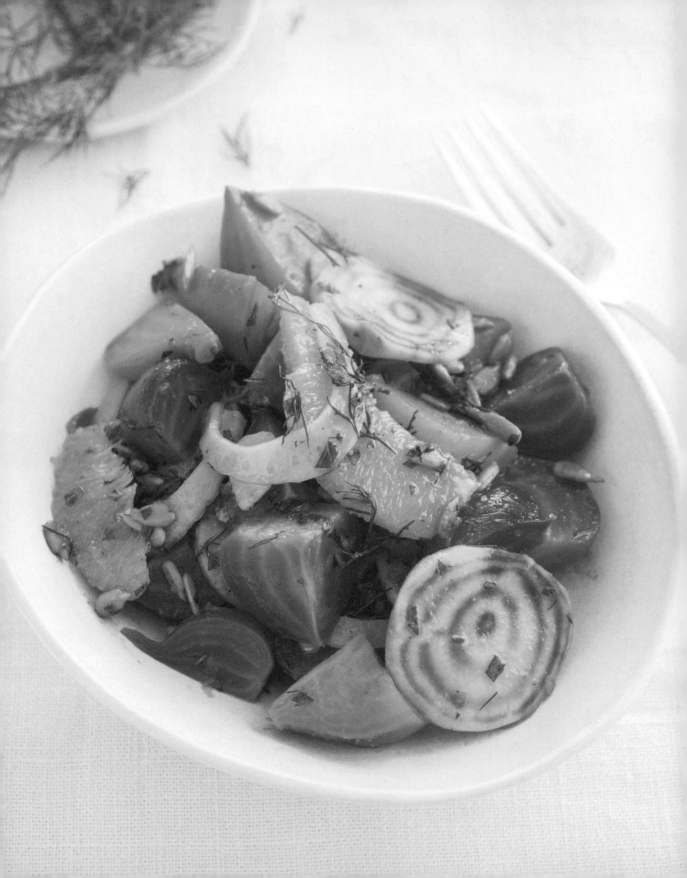

Beet Salad with Fennel, Orange, + Sunflower Gremolata

From Franklin Becker, chef/owner of The Little Beet, New York City

Vegetarian, vegan, dairy-free, gluten-free, nut-free

Beets are one of the best sources of folate, a nutrient that lowers your blood levels of homocysteine, an inflammatory amino acid. Combined with vitamin C-rich oranges, which protect your skin from environmental stressors, and vitamin E-dense sunflower seeds, which help your body heal from within, this salad will keep the color on your plate—and off your face!

Serves 4

1 bunch baby golden beets, roasted

1 bunch baby red beets, roasted

4 tablespoons extra-virgin olive oil, divided

Salt, to taste

Pepper, to taste

1 tablespoon sherry vinegar

1 tablespoon honey

1 teaspoon Dijon mustard

1 bunch raw baby candy-striped beets

3 tablespoons sunflower seeds, toasted

2 teaspoons Maldon sea salt flakes

¼ teaspoon cayenne pepper

1 tablespoon parsley leaves

1 tablespoon dill

1 tablespoon mint leaves

1 tablespoon chervil

1 teaspoon lemon zest

1 teaspoon orange zest

1 small fennel bulb, thinly sliced

1 orange, sectioned

Preheat the oven to 350°F.

Toss the golden and red beets with 3 tablespoons oil, salt, and pepper and wrap separately in tin foil. Bake until fork-tender, about 30 minutes.

Remove from the oven and peel the beets, while still hot, under cool running water. Quarter the beets and toss with vinegar, honey, and mustard. Marinate for 1 hour.

Peel and thinly slice the baby candy-striped beets on a mandolin. Set aside.

In a mixing bowl, combine the toasted sunflower seeds, sea salt, cayenne pepper, parsley, dill, mint, chervil, lemon zest, orange zest, and 1 tablespoon of oil.

Toss with all of the beets and sliced fennel immediately prior to serving.

Top with orange sections.

Lemon Berry Parfait

From Cassandra Shupp, pastry chef at Topping Rose House, Bridgehampton, NY
Vegetarian, vegan, dairy-free, gluten-free, nut-free

Cooling your body temperature will help to mute facial flushing, which is just one reason I love this lemon berry parfait recipe. The other reason (beyond it being delicious) is that with so many antioxidant-packed berries, this parfait will also help to protect your skin from further environmental damage, which can lead to further flare-ups whether your redness is caused by rosacea, acne, sun damage, a rash, or anything else.

Serves 4

LEMON SORBET

3 ½ cups white sugar

4 ½ cups water, divided

2 lemons, zested

2 cups lemon juice

BERRY SAUCE

¼ cup blueberries

¼ cup raspberries

¼ cup blackberries

¼ cup sugar

8 tablespoons framboise (raspberry) lambic beer (optional)

FRESH BERRY SALAD

Small bunch of fresh basil leaves

½ cup blueberries

½ cup raspberries

½ cup blackberries

½ teaspoon lemon juice

2 tablespoons berry sauce

For the Lemon Sorbet

Combine the sugar, 2⅔ cups water, and lemon zest in a pot and bring to a boil. In a separate bowl, combine lemon juice and remaining water.

Once the sugar mixture begins to boil, pour it into the lemon juice mixture and let it cool to room temperature.

Strain out the zest and freeze until it starts to solidify, then pull out and scrape about every hour.

For the Berry Sauce

Cook the berries and the sugar over medium-high heat until they start to break down and a sauce begins to form. Continue cooking berries, stirring occasionally, until the berries begin to thicken.

Add in the lambic beer, if desired, and turn heat down to a medium-low heat. Stir until berries are completely broken down and a thick sauce has formed.

Strain out the seeds and let it cool to room temperature.

For the Fresh Berry Salad

Layer a few basil leaves on top of each other, rolling together into a log, and cut into thin strips. Toss all ingredients until the berries are lightly coated and glisten with sauce.

In a short-stemmed coupe glass, add a little of the berry sauce and fresh berry salad to the bottom of the coupe. Layer two scoops of the lemon sorbet on top. Sprinkle more of the berry salad over top and add a third scoop of lemon sorbet over that. Top with a splash of lambic, if desired, for an extra kick and added bubbles. Garnish with the bud of the basil stem and additional berry sauce, as desired.

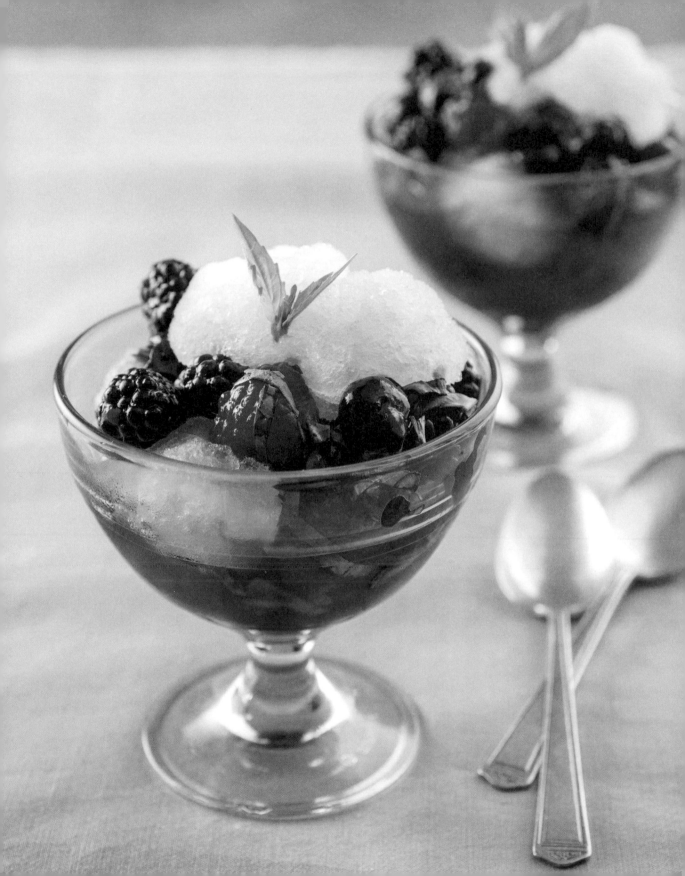

Dull, Dry, Drab Skin

Just like your fuel-burning metabolism slows as you age, so too does your skin's metabolism. As we get older (even in our twenties), our skin both creates new cells and sheds the old ones more slowly. The result: a built-up layer of dead and dull skin cells sitting on the surface of your face, giving you the appearance of an ashy, vampire-like complexion (without the allure of a *Twilight* saga).

Retinols and chemical peels are so effective in making our skin glow because in causing your body to shed those dead, dull skin cells, they reveal the youthful, new skin cells underneath. The side effects, however—namely chapped, red skin that sheds like a snake—aren't pretty. And why slather on chemicals when there are other natural options? Hey, if a skincare product isn't approved for use on pregnant women because of its potential effects on an unborn baby, you may not want it on or in your body either, right?

Thankfully, staying chemical-free doesn't mean you're destined to have dull skin. Rather, retinols get their power from vitamin A—the same vitamin A found in the produce aisle. And chemical peels are derived from acids—like the lactic acid found in milk and citric acid found in fruits. So why not skip the chemicals and instead meet me in the kitchen?

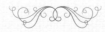

Apply

DIY Beauty Cures for Dull, Dry, Drab Skin

When it comes to revealing a more hydrated, luminous complexion, the key is two-fold. First is getting rid of the dead, dull skin cells concealing your skin's true radiance. Second is applying moisturizing agents, which without prior exfoliating, merely sit on the surface of your skin, unable to penetrate.

While manual exfoliators (like those granular scrubs you buy at the drugstore) can get the job done, those rough beads often tear your skin at the cellular level, leaving you more prone to the effects of aging later on. The secret is to first chemically loosen the dull skin cells before gently exfoliating them away—it's why all of the APPLY recipes here require the recipe to first sit on your skin before scrubbing it away.

Avocado + Oatmeal
Revival Mask

Sensitive skin

While sugar and salt scrubs are great for your body, they can be a bit too rough for your sensitive facial skin. That doesn't mean that your face is destined to remain dull and drab though. With ground oats, this gentle mask calms as it exfoliates, while simultaneously moisturizing with avocado's abundant fatty acids, so you can rest assured that your sensitive skin is exfoliated, not irritated.

¼ cup oatmeal

1 avocado

2 tablespoons honey

In a food processor, grind oatmeal until sand-like. Transfer to a small bowl.

In the same food processor, purée avocado and honey until smooth.

Mix oats with avocado and honey until well combined.

Apply a thin layer to your face and neck and let it sit for 15 to 20 minutes.

Cover your face with a warm washcloth for an additional 3 to 5 minutes to soften the mask and encourage the avocado oil to penetrate more deeply.

Use the washcloth to gently remove the mask, using a circular, upward motion.

Quick Tips

• Cut a red grape in half and rub the flat side on your skin. Grapes contain glucose, which hydrates your skin, as well as anti-aging antioxidants!

• If you want to throw your moisturizer into high gear, mix a drop of raw honey into your cream before applying to help the hydrating benefits penetrate more deeply.

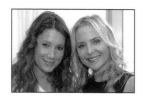

"Just take a handful of white sugar in the shower and scrub! It's the best exfoliator there is. If you look at most exfoliants, it's usually sugar anyway, so why even bother?"

—**Carmindy, makeup artist and host of** *What Not to Wear*

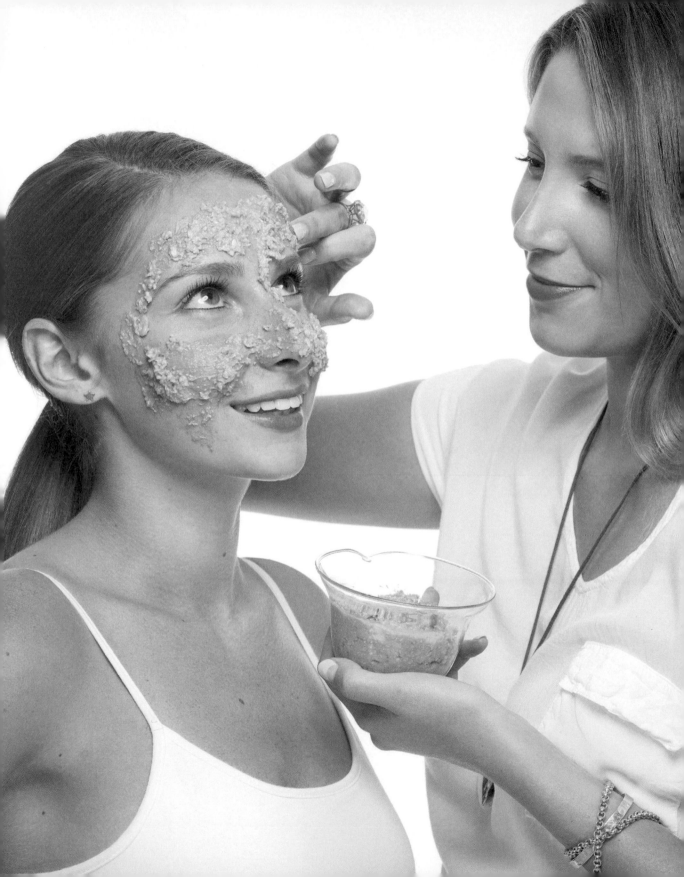

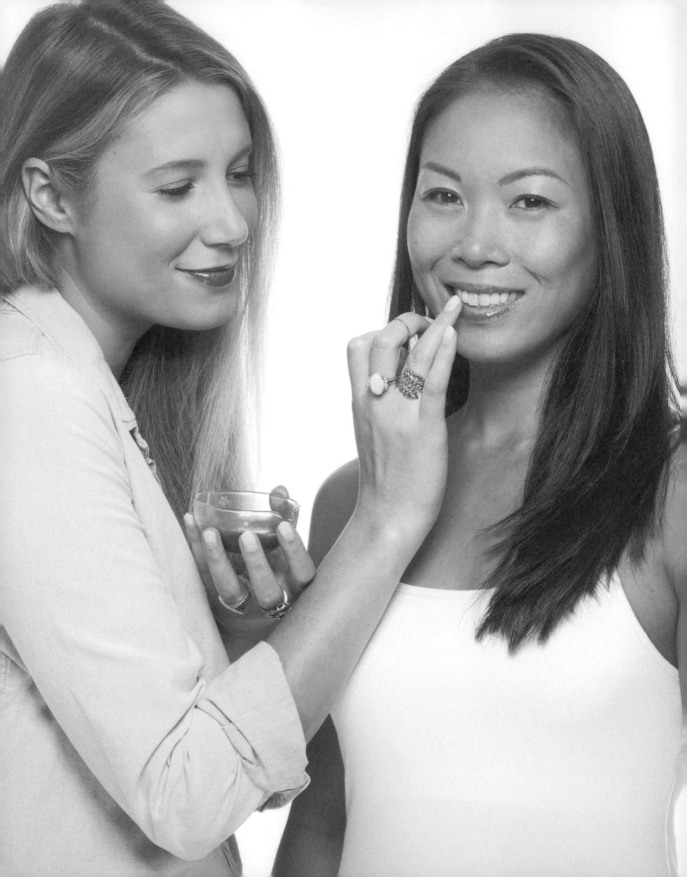

Sweet Lip Scrub

From Frances Hathaway, celebrity makeup artist

All skin types

Want to know how Fergie's lips look so luscious? Make-up artist Frances Hathaway, who uses this brown sugar and honey lip scrub on models and celebrities all the time, used it on Fergie at the shoot of her fragrance campaign. She says, "Just a little bit of brown sugar and honey makes a moisturizing exfoliating lip scrub in a pinch. Mix it together, let it sit, and rub it off before applying lipstick." Since Frances gave me that tip I've used it often—and, not just because I want to be just a wee bit more like Fergie (and marrying Josh Duhamel is off the table).

1 teaspoon honey
1 teaspoon brown sugar

Mix the honey and sugar together before applying a thick layer to your lips.

Let it sit for 5 minutes before using your finger to scrub away softened skin.

Remove excess with a damp washcloth before applying lipstick.

Strawberry + Kiwi Fruit Peel

Sun-damaged, aging skin

Think of this as an all-natural take on a tradtional chemical peel, without the need for a "don't leave the house" calendar alert (trust me, chemical peels are no joke . . . they're an occupational hazard). With both strawberries and kiwi, this mask's topical vitamin C is ideal for evening out skin tone and fighting free-radical damage, while the smooth little beads of seeds in the kiwi and the smaller, more granular seeds on the strawberries are perfect for gently exfoliating loosened skin cells.

2 to 3 medium strawberries, destemmed
1 kiwi, peeled
1 teaspoon lemon juice

Use a fork to gently mash the strawberries and kiwi before mixing in the lemon juice. Avoid using a blender, which can break down the seeds, which we want to keep intact.

Apply a thick layer to your face and chest, avoiding your eye area.

Let it sit for 10 minutes before rinsing with warm water.

Follow with moisturizer, as desired.

Quick Tip
• Always apply moisturizer to damp skin for maximum hydration.

Pumpkin +
Coconut Gommage

Acne-prone, oily, and aging skin

Reveal a brighter, more youthful complexion and help to deeply hydrate your skin with this all-natural scrub. It contains pumpkin to chemically exfoliate with vitamin A; coconut oil and honey to moisturize; and walnuts and flaxseeds to manually exfoliate. And because honey and coconut oil are both antibacterial, you don't have to worry about this scrub clogging your pores, making it ideal for acne-prone skin that's also looking dull or feeling dry.

2 tablespoons raw walnuts

2 tablespoons pumpkin, fresh and puréed or canned

1 teaspoon extra-virgin cold-pressed coconut oil

1 teaspoon raw honey

2 tablespoons ground flaxseeds

In a food processor, grind the walnuts. (If your skin is sensitive, grind until sand-like. If your skin is less sensitive, grind until the size of small pebbles.)

Mix pumpkin, coconut oil, and honey until well combined. Fold in flaxseeds and ground walnuts.

Apply a thick layer to clean skin and let it sit for 10 minutes before gently scrubbing in upward, circular motions.

Rinse with warm water, allowing residual coconut oil to remain on your skin for its moisturizing benefits.

"A drop of olive oil and a little packet of white sugar and you can exfoliate your lips—follow with any moisturizer, or a dab of honey, to heal chapped lips."

—Robert Verdi, style expert

"I took a tip from Jessica Alba and sometimes create my own peppermint tea toner. It's easy to make, awakens dull skin, and soothes my mind. Brew a bag of peppermint tea and let it cool. Pour the tea into a spray bottle and refrigerate. I use it in the morning before applying moisturizer and throughout the day as a pick-me-up."

—Jeannine Morris, BeautySweetSpot.com

"After I had been traveling loads for *So You Think You Can Dance*, my facialist told me to put olive oil on my skin and I really like it! After I cleanse and wash and before moisturizer I put on a few drops. I look like a giant grease ball but it works—I do it at the airport before a flight too!"

—Cat Deely, TV host

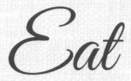

Eat

Food Cures for
Dull, Dry, Drab Skin

If there is one beauty concern for which a change in your diet can provide an *almost* immediate result, it's with regard to dry, dull skin. As your body's largest organ (yup, I said it . . . again!) and certainly the most visible one, your skin is one of the first places to show signs of dehydration. With water making up 60–65 percent of our bodies, just a mild bout of hardly noticeable dehydration—the kind that barely even registers as thirst—can take our complexions from dewy to drab, fast. Unfortunately, chugging some good old H_2O doesn't always cut it—although it's most definitely encouraged. Instead, you need a cocktail of the right vitamins, minerals, fats, and fatty-acids—all of which you'll find here.

Tropical Crab Salad

Dairy-free, gluten-free, nut-free

With water-dense cucumber, beta-carotene-packed mango, healthy fat-filled avocado, and omega-3 fatty acid-rich crab, this salad is to your skin what a canteen filled with purified water is to an explorer lost in the desert: hydrating in the most epic way possible. Plus, it's tropically delicious.

Serves 2

1 English cucumber

1 mango, peeled

1 avocado

1 tablespoon lime juice

Pinch of coarse sea salt

Pinch of cayenne pepper

6 ounces jumbo lump crab meat, divided

Lime slices, to garnish

Chop the cucumber, mango, and avocado into bite-size cubes. Gently toss with the lime juice, salt, and cayenne.

Divide in half before topping each serving with 3 ounces of the jumbo lump crabmeat and garnishing with the lime slices.

Raw Green Soup

Vegetarian, vegan, dairy-free, gluten-free, nut-free

A hybrid of gazpacho and green juice, this creamy (but dairy-free) chilled green soup is an anti-aging elixir of epic proportions. Kiwis, loaded with vitamin C and antioxidants, help to keep skin firm, while avocados and cucumbers help to keep skin hydrated and supple from the inside out. Serve this soup in shot glasses at your next cocktail party, or throw it in a Thermos for a chilled anti-aging soup on the go!

Serves 2

1 kiwi, whole with skin

1 avocado

1 English cucumber, roughly chopped

2 garlic cloves

½ lime, peeled

2 tablespoons chopped cilantro, divided

Jalapeño pepper, sliced, to taste

In a blender, purée the kiwi, avocado, cucumber, garlic, lime, and 1 tablespoon cilantro. Add small slices of jalapeño one by one, to taste.

Refrigerate 2 to 4 hours to chill.

Garnish with additional cilantro prior to serving.

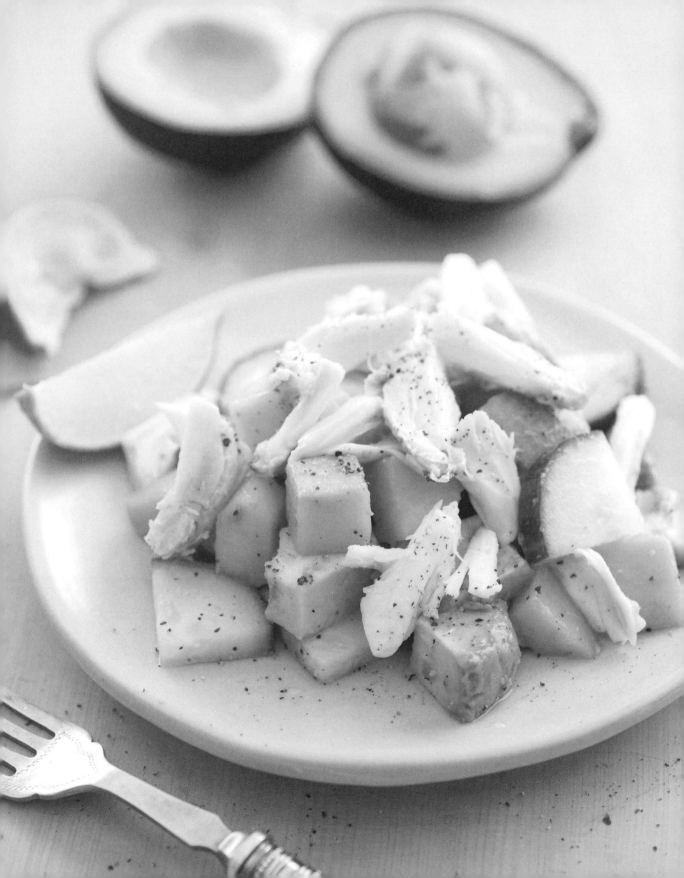

Wild Strawberries + "Top of the Waldorf Rooftop Honey"-Infused Yogurt

From the Waldorf-Astoria Hotel, New York City

Vegetarian, gluten-free, nut-free

Want to know the secret to supple, dewy skin? Just one cup of yummy strawberries packs in more than 150 percent of the recommended daily allowance of the anti-aging super vitamin, vitamin C (more than that found in a serving of oranges or grapefruits), and research shows that people who eat a diet high in vitamin C have less age-related dry skin and even fewer wrinkles than those who don't.

Serves 10

3 pints strawberries

1 cup honey

1 cup plain Greek yogurt

1 tablespoon mint leaves

Wash the strawberries and clip the stems. Leave a small amount of stem to use for dipping into yogurt.

Combine the honey and yogurt and reserve in the refrigerator until ready to serve.

Cut the mint leaves into chiffonade (fine julienne) and toss with the cleaned strawberries. Reserve in the refrigerator until ready to serve.

Serve the strawberries slightly chilled with the yogurt as a dipping sauce.

At the Waldorf-Astoria New York they use their own homegrown "Top of the Waldorf Rooftop Honey."

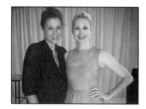

Quick Tip

• Do your teeth need a scrubbing as much as your lips? *Gossip Girl*'s Kelly Rutherford told me she always keeps apples around. A few bites and the combination of the acids and chewing action scrubs her teeth clean when there is no toothbrush in sight!

Protein Crackers with Avocado

Vegetarian, dairy-free, gluten-free

Moisturize dry skin from the inside out with a diet rich in heart-healthy fats like those found in nuts, seeds, and avocados. A take on the traditional English "avocado toast" recipe, this version is low-carb, packed with protein, and loaded with heart-healthy and skin-hydrating fats.

Serves 4 to 6

½ cup raw almonds

½ cup raw cashews

⅓ cup raw pistachios

⅓ cup raw walnuts

⅓ cup raw pumpkin seeds

2 tablespoons raw ground flaxseeds

1 egg

1 teaspoon sea salt

1 tablespoon sesame seeds

1 avocado, sliced

1 tablespoon lemon juice

Red chili flakes, to taste

Preheat the oven to 350°F.

In a food processor, blend the almonds, cashews, pistachios, walnuts, pumpkin seeds, and flaxseeds until powdered.

In a small bowl, mix the nut mixture with the egg, salt, and 2 tablespoons filtered water until it forms a dough.

On a parchment-lined baking sheet, use a spatula to spread the dough into a thin layer, approximately ¼-inch thick. Use a knife to score 3 to 4-inch squares. Around the edges of the dough, use your knife to push in the ends to prevent burning. Sprinkle with water and top with sesame seeds.

Bake for 25 to 30 minutes, watching carefully to ensure they don't burn.

In a small bowl, mash the avocado with the lemon juice. When the crackers are cooled, break apart and top with a dollop of the avocado and sprinkle with chili flakes, to taste.

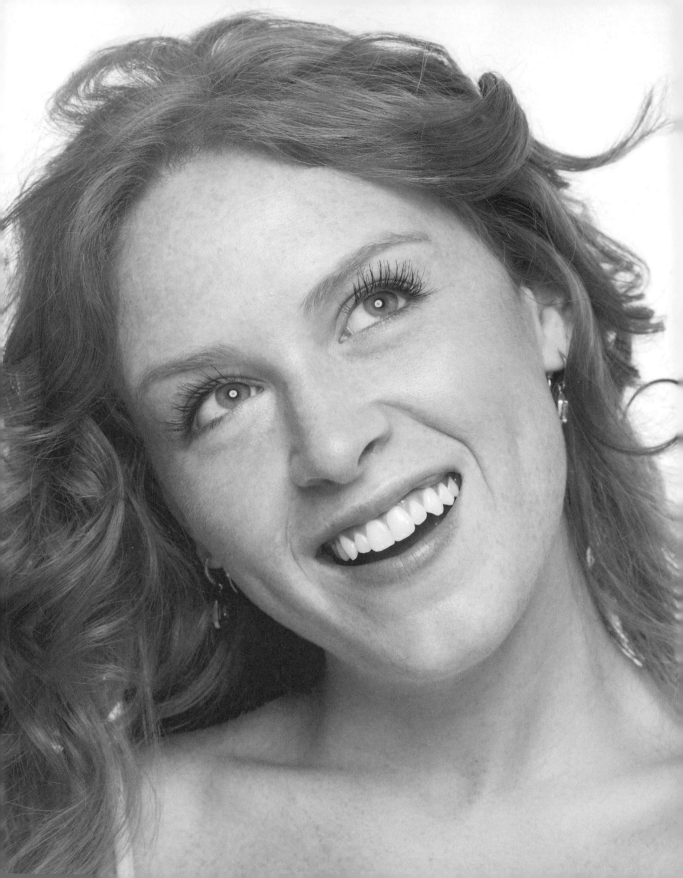

chapter 2
Eyes

Under-eye Circles

If you're like most women, you wake up some mornings with bags under your eyes so big they make the oversized luggage I only seem to spot in the international terminal look like change purses. Sure, a day at the spa and a full eight hours of sleep would do the trick, but who has the time—or the money? And, let's be honest, adding to that credit card debt will only stress you out even more, leading to further sleep deprivation and even bigger under-eye circles than you started with.

Sound familiar? Rather than investing in pricey de-puffing eye gels and circle-reducing eye creams—few of which actually are the miracle workers they claim to be—or buying stock in YSL's Touche Éclat, find a solution in the following pages. Those love handles may not melt away (hey, your body is beautiful just the way it is!), but those under-eye bags will certainly be a thing of the past!

Apply

DIY Beauty Cures
for Under-eye Circles

Just because you wake up with puffy, darkened eyes, doesn't mean you're destined to carry those bags around with you all day—heck, you're likely carrying enough in that purse of yours already! Rather than merely concealing your under-eye circles though, eliminate them (or, at the very least, seriously minimize them) without having to go any further than your refrigerator.

Addressing both dark circles and water retention, these beauty recipes will ensure you're bright-eyed for your day ahead. And, with full awareness that the skin around your eyes is some of the thinnest on your body, you can rest assured that only the healthiest of ingredients are getting close to those precious peepers of yours.

Perk-Up Potato Packs

Not for sensitive skin

Cucumber under-eye compresses may be the more spa-like option, but cucumbers don't get to the root cause of under-eye circles like white potatoes do. Catecholase, an enzyme found in potatoes, is commonly used in high-end skin-care and makeup products as a way to lighten skin and diminish dark eye circles. But why pay for a pricey cream when you can DIY it with potatoes at home? Use refrigerated potatoes and these compresses will simultaneously constrict the blood vessels under your eyes and reduce puffiness and darkness.

1 small Idaho potato
2 cheesecloths

Grate the potato using either a cheese grater or food processor. Wrap ¼ cup of the grated potato in each of the cheesecloths. Tie the ends with a hair elastic or rubber band. Apply as compresses over your eyes for 15 to 20 minutes.

Note: Tight on time? Thin slices of raw potato over your eyes can do the trick, too!

Egg-cellent Eye Gel

All skin types

Next time you make eggs for breakfast, don't toss the eggshells so quickly. Instead, use the remaining egg whites lining the shell to tighten the skin around your eyes, not only reducing puffiness, but also temporarily reducing the appearance of fine lines and wrinkles. Just a thin layer of the gel-like egg whites dries to firm fine lines and wrinkles while simultaneously hydrating tired eyes and reducing the appearance of under-eye puffiness. The effects are temporary, but the results speak for themselves—especially before a big event or on a morning when it seems as if those crow's feet had a bit of a growth spurt overnight.

1 egg white, raw (or a leftover shell)

After cracking an egg, wipe your finger along the inside of the shell.

Dab a thick layer of the raw egg white under and around your eye, avoiding the eyelid and being careful not to get raw egg in your eye.

Let the egg white fully dry, about 15 minutes, before rinsing off with lukewarm water. Follow with eye cream, if desired.

Note: While I recommend leaving the egg whites on for about 15 minutes before rinsing with luke-warm water, if you apply a thin enough layer, you can leave the mask on all day underneath your eye makeup. Just be careful to check sporadically for unfortunate cracks. That's never a good look!

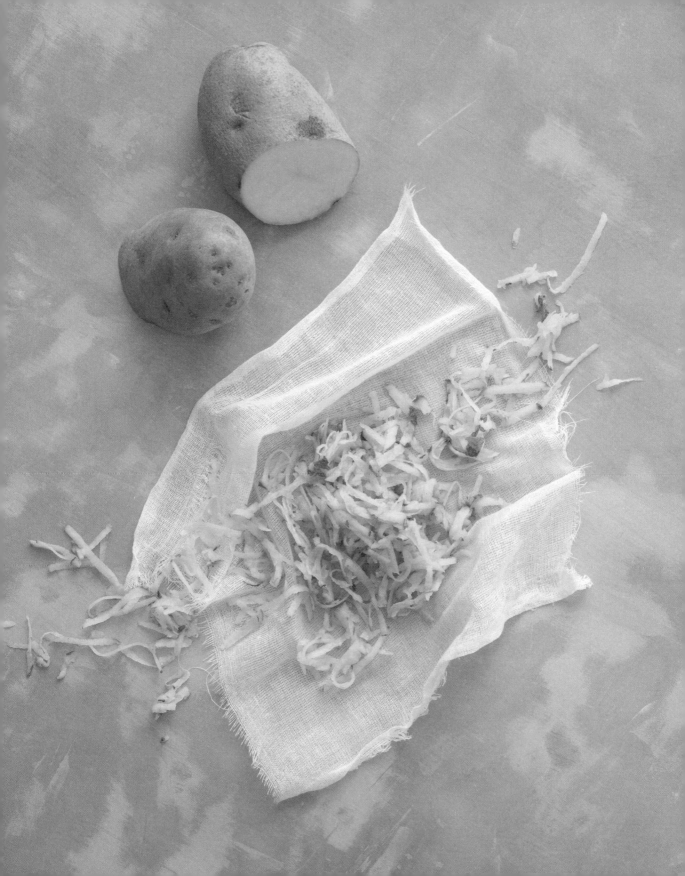

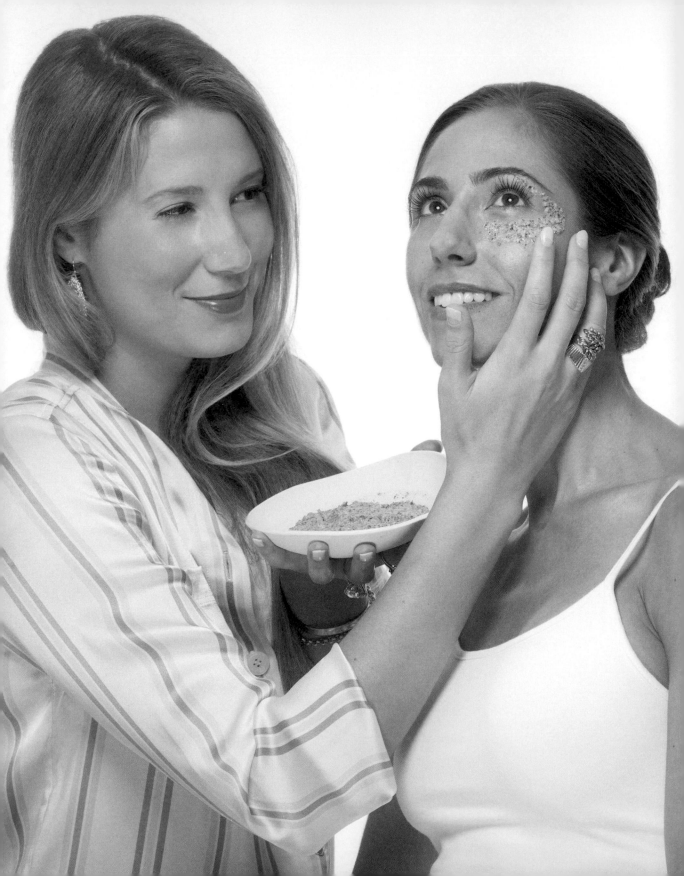

Faux-Rested Eye Mask

All skin types

Need to look well rested in a dash? A pinch of parsley can do the trick. It's rich in vitamin K, which may as well be called the "eye-opening vitamin," both in your diet and in your skincare. Parsley, when applied topically, helps to reduce blood flow to the under-eye area, diminishing the appearance of underlying blood vessels. This is an especially useful trick as we age and the fat deposits under our eyes thin, making blood vessels even more visible. Blended with cooling and hydrating cucumber to plump and de-puff and deeply moisturizing and gently exfoliating yogurt, this eye mask should become a staple in your fridge. As an added bonus, mixed with lemon juice, it doubles as a delicious salad dressing, too.

1 tablespoon plain full-fat Greek yogurt
1 tablespoon minced parsley
1 cucumber slice, 1-inch thick

Place the yogurt, parsley, and cucumber in a food processor and pulse until a smooth paste forms.

Apply a thick layer under your eyes and on your brow bone, avoiding your eyelid where the skin is too thin and being careful not to get the mixture in your eye.

Let it sit for 20 minutes before removing excess with a cotton ball or washcloth and rinsing any remaining residue off with cool water.

Quick Tip
• Use an under-eye concealer with yellow undertones for better coverage.

Iced Tea Toner

All skin types

Two of the best cures for dark under-eye circles are caffeine and cold. I'm not talking about chugging an iced coffee. I'm talking about both applying caffeine and cooling your eyes, topically, with this homemade iced tea toner. For a quick, easy, and highly effective trick, make caffeinated ice cubes with black tea to get rid of under-eye darkness and puffiness, naturally and affordably!

2 cups water
4 bags caffeinated black tea

Bring the water to a boil. Reduce to a simmer and place the tea bags in the water to brew for 15 to 20 minutes.

Remove it from the heat and let it sit until the tea cools to room temperature.

Once cool, pour the brew into ice cube trays and freeze overnight.

In the morning, pop out two of the cubes and run them under water for a second to wet the surface and prevent it from sticking to your skin.

Gently rub under your eyes for 1 to 2 minutes.

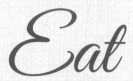

Eat

Food Cures
for Under-eye Circles

If under-eye circles have you down and extra shut-eye isn't cutting it (or isn't possible), consider this: under-eye puffiness and darkness are often caused by nutritional deficiencies—meaning that no matter how early your hit the sack or how many topical beauty recipes you whip up, you may never banish the burden of that under-eye baggage unless you change your diet.

So, how do you eat for rested eyes? Load up on vitamin K, which is essential for normal clotting and blood flow in our bodies, including under our eyes; iron, which helps carry oxygen through your body to make you feel and look strong and awake; and B vitamins, which are important for energy. Deficiencies in any these impact circulation and, therefore, affect how perky we look and feel.

Garden Vegetable Omelet

Vegetarian, gluten-free, nut-free

You may think hitting the snooze button for an extra (not-so-helpful) ten minutes of sleep is a good way to minimize under-eye circles, but what if I told you getting up a bit earlier and making this delicious breakfast is actually the secret not only to yummier mornings but to looking more rested, too? This eye-opening omelet is loaded with under-eye-bag banishing peas and carrots, which are rich in vitamin K, and eggs, which are packed with iron. When added to your regular morning routine, it will perk up tired eyes. Literally.

Serves 1 to 2

¼ cup peas (fresh or frozen)

¼ cup diced carrots (fresh or frozen)

¼ cup chopped broccoli (fresh or frozen)

¼ cup corn (fresh or frozen)

2 tablespoons extra-virgin olive oil

3 eggs

Pinch of salt

Ground black pepper, to taste

2 tablespoons shredded Cheddar cheese (optional)

Sauté the peas, carrots, broccoli, and corn in the oil, over medium heat, until tender.

In a small bowl, beat the eggs and season with the salt and pepper.

If you're using frozen vegetables, drain the water that has accumulated in the bottom of the pan.

Pour the eggs over the vegetables, gently stirring the mixture using a heat-resistant spatula to ensure they're evenly distributed.

Reduce heat and continue cooking for about 1 to 2 minutes. The eggs should appear cooked toward the edges, but runny on top.

Flip the omelet and sprinkle with the cheese, if desired. Cover for 1 to 2 minutes before removing from the heat and folding the omelet in half.

Top with fresh ground pepper, to taste.

Quick Tips

• Keep iron-rich breakfast cereals at your desk to munch away under-eye circles throughout the day.

• Under-eye circles can be a sign of anemia, a more severe iron deficiency that requires medical attention. If you are feeling tired, weak, cold, short of breath, or displaying any other symptoms, check with your doctor.

"Anything cold, be it cucumbers, frozen peas, or the backside of a cold spoon will help a tired eye."
    —Lauren Conrad, author and TV personality

Coffee Rubbed Chicken + Farro Salad

From Karen Nicolas, *Food & Wine* magazine's Best New Chef, 2012

Dairy-free

The caffeine in the coffee rub on this chicken may help you feel more awake, but it's not the only reason this recipe will help reduce the appearance of under-eye circles. Farro, with its fiber, protein, magnesium, and B vitamins, and iron-rich chicken, can help you feel energized—and look it, too—by increasing both skin hydration and circulation.

Serves 4

COFFEE RUBBED CHICKEN

½ cup ground espresso beans

¼ cup chili powder

¼ cup ground coriander seeds

¼ cup packed dark brown sugar

¼ cup cocoa powder

2 tablespoons dry mustard powder

2 tablespoons salt

1 tablespoon ground black peppercorn

3 tablespoons extra virgin olive oil

4 boneless chicken breasts

FARRO SALAD

1 cup dry farro

¾ cup chopped onion

2 tablespoons chopped rosemary sprigs

1 teaspoon ground coriander

1 cinnamon stick

2½ cups chicken or vegetable stock

2 summer plums, sliced into 8 wedges

1 cup toasted walnuts, roughly chopped

¼ cup sherry wine vinegar

2 tablespoons red wine vinegar

2 tablespoons Dijon mustard

¾ cups extra-virgin olive oil

2 tablespoons walnut oil

Salt, to taste

Black peppercorn, to taste

For the Coffee Rubbed Chicken

Preheat the oven to 350°F.

In a mixing bowl, combine all of the dry ingredients.

Season the chicken breasts liberally with the coffee rub.

Heat a large sauté pan over a medium flame. Once the pan is hot, add the oil to the pan. Sear the chicken for 2 minutes on each side to toast the spices.

Place the chicken in a baking pan and bake at 350°F until the chicken is cooked all the way through, about 12 minutes.

For the Farro Salad

Place the farro in a colander and rinse it through running water to clean.

Sweat the onions in a medium sauce pot, until tender.

Add the farro, rosemary, coriander, and cinnamon stick and cook until the farro is slightly toasted, about 2 minutes.

Add the stock and simmer until the farro is tender.

Strain the farro of any excess liquid before seasoning with salt and peppercorn. Allow the farro to cool to room temperature.

Toss the farro with the sliced plums and walnuts.

In a mixing bowl, combine the vinegars and mustard with a whisk. Slowly whisk in the oils to create an emulsion.

Season with the salt and peppercorn.

Add the vinegar mixture to the farro.

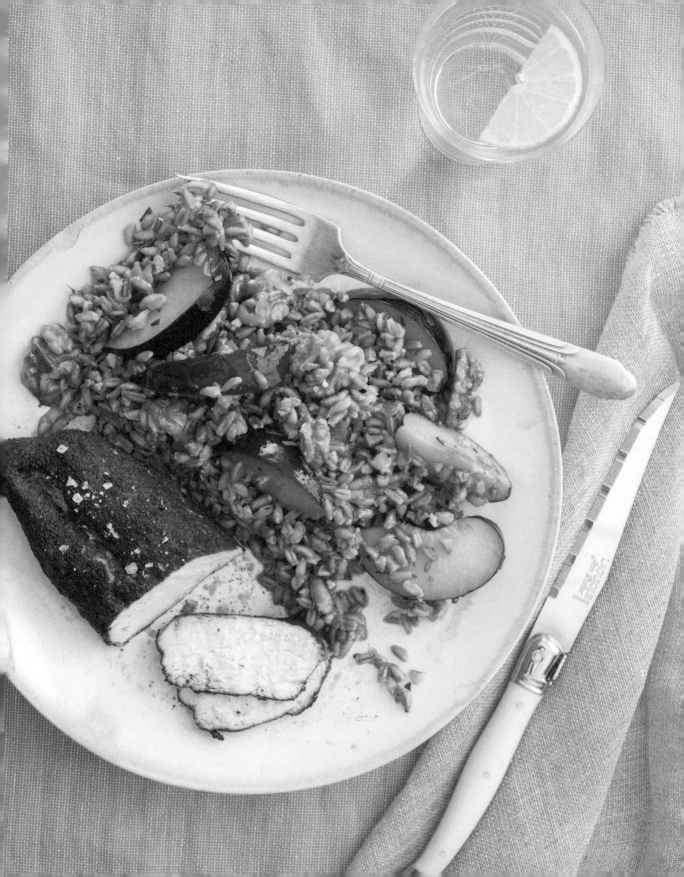

Creamy Kale + Walnut Salad

Vegetarian, vegan, dairy-free, gluten-free

Kale tops the "rich in vitamin K" charts, making this salad just what your under-eye circles need to hibernate for good. For good measure, top this creamy kale salad with walnuts, which not only add a toasted crunch, but also are a good source of sleep-promoting melatonin. That'll make sure this salad works double duty on your sleep-deprived eyes when you have it for dinner.

Serves 2

3 tablespoons raw walnuts

½ ripe avocado

2 teaspoons extra-virgin olive oil

Salt, to taste

8 stems kale, chopped

2 fillets (4 ounces) salmon or chicken breasts, grilled (optional)

Toast the raw walnuts in a dry skillet until slightly browned, about 2 minutes, watching carefully to make sure they don't burn.

Mash the avocado with the oil and salt to form a creamy dressing.

Use your hands to massage the chopped kale leaves with the avocado mixture until tender.

Top with the toasted walnuts and either grilled salmon or chicken, if desired.

Quick Tips

• Dairy, wheat, and other common food allergies can cause puffiness and discoloration to your under-eye area. If your problem persists, check with your doctor about allergy testing.

• Double up on your pillows. By keeping your head slightly elevated, you will reduce the amount of fluid that accumulates underneath your eyes and reduce under-eye puffiness.

• Get moving! Even if you're time strapped, try doing some jumping jacks, squats, or pushups in the morning to help get your heart rate up. By increasing your heart rate, you improve your body's circulation, which helps not only increase your energy level but also reduces under-eye bags and circles.

• Use under eye creams with a slight shimmer to reflect the light and reduce the appearance of under-eye darkness—although be forewarned that shimmer can settle in fine lines and wrinkles, making them appear more pronounced.

"My eyes are very sensitive so I put spoons in the freezer and then place the frozen spoons on my eyes when they're irritated or when I'm tired."

—Whitney Port, fashion designer and TV personality

Smile Lines, Crow's Feet, + Other Eye Wrinkle Euphemisms

When it comes to the first signs of aging, for most of us the eye area is where it's at. And not in a good way.

Sure, fine lines in the corners of your eyes are indicators of a life well laughed, but that doesn't mean they're a welcome addition to our faces, or that they're inevitable. Heck, BO is a sign of a great workout, but that doesn't mean that anyone wants to walk around stinking up the place in the name of proving their sweaty success.

As the thinnest skin on your body, the area around your eyes is very absorbent, very sensitive, and very reactive. This means that all-natural, homemade beauty recipes are the ideal remedy for wrinkles around the eyes because the last thing you want to do is saturate the area with chemicals. Anything too strong (even my all natural anti-aging remedies designed for the rest of your face) can cause more harm than good to this delicate area.

If you're primarily concerned with fine lines on the outer corners of your eyes or creeping underneath, if you're looking to mitigate the wrinkling that's already begun or stave off the fine lines you know are en route, these homemade recipes are the best way to treat your concerns. Eyes may be the windows to the soul, as they say, but they don't have to reveal our age, too!

Apply

DIY Beauty Cures for Smile Lines, Crow's Feet, + Other Eye Wrinkle Euphemisms

Women ask me all the time about when they should start an anti-aging regimen and my go-to answer is usually, "If you're old enough to know what one is, you should probably be on it." But that doesn't mean you need to go out and spend a small fortune on pricey anti-aging cleansers, serums, and creams.

Whether your eyes are already showing signs of a life well-lived or you're just looking to prevent the signs from showing up for quite some time, try out these all natural remedies. With potent doses of active ingredients and without any nasty preservatives, the anti-aging benefits in homemade beauty recipes are able to penetrate deeply for a fraction of the price and without the risk of chemicals permeating and irritating your skin.

Just remember, while these under-eye beauty recipes are safe for the rest of your face, the reverse is not always true, so don't apply skincare products or other DIY recipes intended for other parts of the body to the delicate area around your eyes.

Two-in-One Anti-Aging
Makeup Remover

All skin types

For many women, one of the only times we pay attention to the area around our eyes is when applying makeup or when removing our eye makeup at the end of the day. In both cases, we're often in a rush, rubbing and tugging away. When we so frequently pull on this delicate area of skin—like when you tug on a rubber band for too long—it loses its elasticity. Only patience and care will keep you from yanking when applying your makeup, but a great eye makeup remover can help keep you from pulling when it's time to take it all off.

After years of struggling to remove waterproof makeup and trying to find an eye makeup remover that didn't irritate, I finally decided to make my own that would break down even the most stubborn eye makeup! As an added bonus: the avocado and coconut oils in this one double as my gently exfoliating and extremely hydrating night eye cream, too!

**1 tablespoon extra-virgin
cold-pressed coconut oil**
1 teaspoon avocado oil

If the coconut oil is solidified (it's a solid at less than 76°F), place the container in a bowl of hot (not boiling) water until melted.

In a small bowl, mix the coconut oil and avocado oil before transferring to a small plastic container. Store in the refrigerator to keep solidified.

To use, warm a small amount in your hands before *gently* massaging around your eyes to emulsify the makeup.

Use a cotton pad or a tissue to gently wipe away the makeup. Repeat until the cotton wipes clean.

Leave residual oil on your skin to penetrate overnight.

Quick Tips
• Apply all these DIY recipes around your lips, too! They will help to prevent the vertical fine lines that make lipstick bleed as you age.

• Don't over-wash your face. Cleansing too often or too aggressively can leave your skin dry and your eyes more wrinkle-prone.

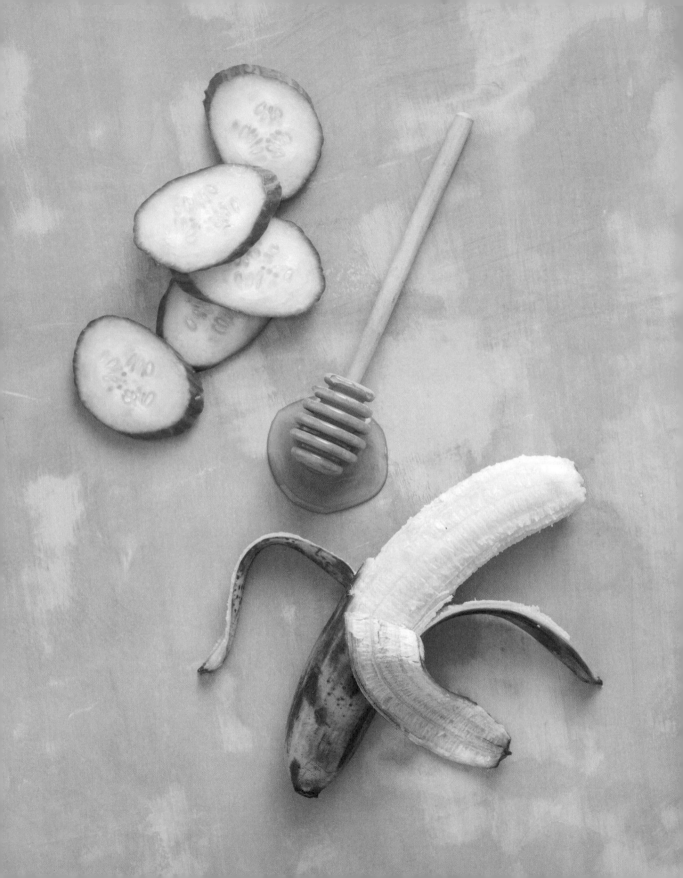

Plump 'Em Up
Eye Mask

All skin types

If you've had a piece of dried fruit recently, you know how wrinkly things get when dehydrated. And because the skin around your eyes is so incredibly thin, it's one of the first areas to lose moisture— and show it. To take your eyes from shriveled up raisin-like to plump and grape-like, use this hydrating under-eye mask. With bananas, rich in potassium, a mineral that helps cells retain their moisture; honey, which helps to gently pull moisture deep below the skin's surface; and cucumbers, with their high water content, this mask is one of the quickest and easiest ways to plump up fine lines.

¼ **ripe banana**

¼ **cucumber, peeled**

1 tablespoon raw honey

Purée all the ingredients in a blender, until smooth. Refrigerate until cool to the touch, about 30 minutes. Apply a thin layer under your eyes and let it sit for 15 minutes before rinsing with warm water.

Quick Tip

• Actress and makeup artist McKenzie Westmore told me that when working on set she pats a thin layer of chilled egg whites under the eyes and lets it dry completely to refresh skin, plump it up, and tighten skin before applying foundation on top for a smooth, refreshed look.

Rejuvenating
Eye Polish

All skin types

As with the rest of your face, exfoliation is essential to any anti-aging routine. When exfoliating around your eyes, though, this needs to be done extremely gently or you risk pulling on the thin, gentle skin, causing more harm than good. Steering clear of aggressive, granular exfoliants in favor of the naturally occurring lactic acid found in milk, this compress gently breaks down dead skin cells to reveal a more youthful complexion. Simultaneously, it hydrates with the fat in both the milk and avocado and protects through the antioxidant-rich grape seed oil.

1 tablespoon avocado
1 tablespoon grape seed oil
3 tablespoons whole milk

Using a fork or a blender, combine the avocado with the grape seed oil until creamy. Slowly add the milk until well combined.

Saturate 2 cotton pads with the mixture and apply under your eyes for 15 minutes.

Rinse with warm water and pat dry.

Quick Tips

• Always apply sunscreen around your eyes and wear sunglasses when outside to protect your skin from wrinkle-causing sun damage.

• Use your ring finger to apply eye creams for the gentlest application.

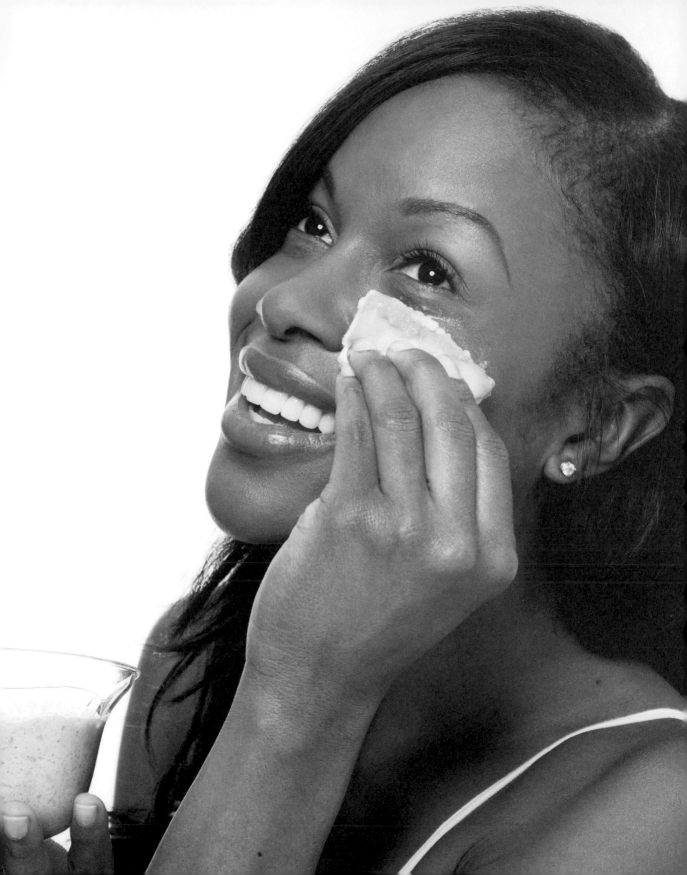

Eat

Food Cures for Smile Lines, Crow's Feet, + Other Eye Wrinkle Euphemisms

Wrinkles around and under your eyes are not merely to be prevented, but also corrected. With a diet rich in antioxidants and omega-3 fatty acids and low in sodium, you can boost your collagen production, ensure that your skin's elasticity is kept intact, and protect yourself from the aging effects of environmental damage. Add in lots of fruit and vegetables, healthy fats, and at least eight glasses of water each day, and your eyes will look younger longer—along with the rest of your body.

Dukkah-Honey Crusted Halibut

From Marissa Lippert, owner of Nourish Kitchen + Table, New York City

Dairy-free, gluten-free

Help skin to maintain its elasticity while also protecting it from future UV damage by loading up on omega-3 fatty acids, like those found in halibut, almonds, hazelnuts, and sesame seeds. Halibut is also a good source of magnesium and B vitamins, which improves circulation.

Not into fish? You can use this same skin-plumping crust recipe with poultry or tofu—or sprinkle it into olive oil as a dipping sauce.

Serves 2

¼ cup raw almonds

¼ cup hazelnuts

2 tablespoons sesame seeds

1 ½ teaspoons cumin seeds

½ teaspoon black peppercorns

2 ½ teaspoons ground coriander

½ teaspoon dried mint

1 teaspoon lemon or orange zest

¼ teaspoon red chili flakes

2 fillets (6 ounces) halibut

Kosher salt, to taste

Extra-virgin olive oil, as needed

2 teaspoons honey

Toast the almonds and hazelnuts in a dry skillet until fragrant. Set aside.

Toast the sesame and cumin seeds in the skillet until fragrant.

Combine the nuts, seeds, and peppercorns in a food processor and pulse until ground. Add in the ground coriander, dried mint, citrus zest, and chili flakes and pulse lightly until blended. Set aside.

Season the halibut with kosher salt and drizzle with the oil. Press each side of the fillet into the spice mix. Drizzle the top of each fillet with the honey.

Heat the oil in a cast-iron pan or oven-proof skillet over medium-high heat. Sear the fish for 3 to 4 minutes on each side.

Finish the fish under the broiler for 1 minute, or until flaky.

Quick Tips

• Get some more Zzz's—a good night's sleep not only helps to reduce the appearance of under-eye circles, but also helps your body to produce more human growth hormone, which helps skin maintain its elasticity!

• Get your eyes checked by an optometrist. By maintaining optimal vision (with the help of glasses or contacts), you'll keep wrinkle-causing squinting at bay.

• Caffeine and sodium can leave you parched, and looking more wrinkled—so keep coffee and salt intake to a minimum to keep your eyes looking as youthful as possible.

• Use organic cotton to remove eye makeup. It's gentle and will help ensure you pull the skin as minimally as possible.

• Snack on raw jicama! The crisp root vegetable boosts collagen production and fights wrinkles, keeping crow's feet away.

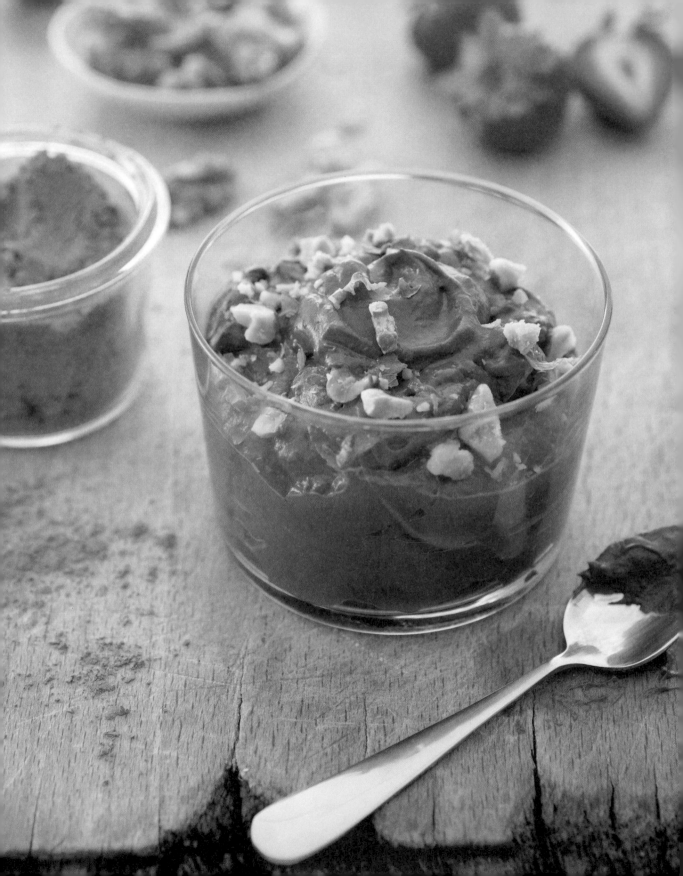

Raw Brownie Batter Pudding

Vegetarian, vegan, dairy-free, gluten-free

Love chocolate? Lucky for you, raw cacao ("nature's chocolate," if you will) is loaded with anti-aging flavonoids, procyanidin, and catechins. Plus, avocado, the base of this raw brownie batter pudding, is packed with hydrating and anti-aging fats and antioxidants that protect skin from sun damage and ensure that skin stays hydrated, supple, and youthful. You can use this as a dip for apples, bananas, or strawberries, too, for a healthier (and anti-aging) take on chocolate covered fruit.

Serves 2
1 ripe avocado
4 tablespoons raw cacao powder

2 tablespoons agave
1 tablespoon vanilla extract
2 tablespoons almond milk, unsweetened
1 tablespoon chopped walnuts (optional)
Granny Smith apple (optional)
Banana (optional)
Strawberries (optional)

Purée the avocado in a food processor or with an immersion blender until creamy.

Slowly add the raw cacao powder, agave, vanilla extract, and almond milk, stirring constantly, until well blended.

Top with walnuts and/or fruit for dipping, if desired. Serve immediately.

Grilled Salmon Salad

From Sonia Kashuk, makeup artist and founder of Sonia Kashuk Beauty
Dairy-free, gluten-free, nut-free

While greens and arugula are great for your health, loaded with vitamins and minerals and packed with antioxidants, the real beauty booster in this fresh and simple salad is the salmon. Packed with protein, salmon improves the production of collagen, keratin, and melanin in your skin, while both helping skin retain water and making you less prone to wrinkles, thanks to its omega-3 fatty acids. As an added bonus: the monounsaturated fat in avocado reduces tissue inflammation and helps your body absorb the fat-soluble vitamins in the greens, all vital for youthful-looking skin and wrinkle-free eyes.

Serves 2
2 cups mixed greens
1 cup arugula
1 avocado, cubed
Extra-virgin olive oil, to taste
Balsamic vinegar, to taste
2 fillets (6 ounces) salmon, grilled

Toss the mixed greens, arugula, and avocado with the oil and the vinegar, to taste. Top with the grilled salmon.

Red, Itchy, Puffy, Bloodshot Eyes

When a bad breakup leaves your eyes red and puffy, allergies leave your peepers bloodshot and itchy, or for whatever other reason, you wake up with irritated and less-than-attractive eyes, there's no need to suffer indefinitely. Sure, a good night's sleep can help if the cause is sleep deprivation, and an allergy pill can help if it's allergies, but when those solutions either aren't available or aren't cutting it, your kitchen can be the key to getting back your bright-eyed gaze. The trick is to calm irritation, alleviate puffiness, and constrict the redness-causing blood vessels—all as quickly as possible.

Whether you are chronically combating bloodshot eyes (did you know your diet could be to blame?!), are a seasonal allergy sufferer (I am, too!), or are just in need of a good cry (we've all been there!), read on to make sure no one's the wiser.

Apply

DIY Beauty Cures for Red, Itchy, Puffy, Bloodshot Eyes

Topical remedies for red, itchy, bloodshot eyes are all about soothing, calming, constricting, and de-puffing. With caffeine, riboflavin, and more, these topical remedies rely on foods like cooling cucumbers, tightening eggs, de-puffing dairy, and anti-inflammatory Indian gooseberry, to take your eyes from red, itchy, bloodshot, and puffy to calm, cool, and collected.

Optic Tea Treatment

All skin types

Black tea, with caffeine to constrict blood vessels and tannins to reduce puffiness, reduces redness, and revives exhausted eyes when applied topically. Add honey to hydrate and soothe and these tea cubes are a quick and easy solution for puffy, red eyes. If you're an allergy sufferer, make a larger batch and keep this in the freezer all season long.

1 cup water
4 bags caffeinated black tea
2 tablespoons honey

Bring water to boil. Remove from heat and add the tea bags.

Steep for 30 minutes, using a spoon to squeeze the tea bags every 10 minutes. Remove the tea bags, again squeezing the bags to extract as much tea as possible.

Stir in the honey.

Pour the mixture into an ice cube tray and freeze.

Once frozen, pop out 2 cubes, run them briefly under water to ensure they're wet and won't stick to your skin, and rub them over and under your eyes for 15 minutes.

Cucumber + Yogurt Cooler

All skin types

Cucumbers are the go-to spa remedy for swollen eyes, and for good reason. Not only are they very hydrating, but with their ascorbic and caffeic acid, they also help to reduce swelling. Paired with whole milk-based yogurt to further constrict blood vessels, de-puff, and hydrate, this soothing mask is one of my tried-and-trusted remedies for reversing the effects of a night spent sniffling (from allergies or tears!).

¼ cup peeled and diced cucumber
¼ cup plain full-fat yogurt

In a blender, purée the cucumber until smooth. Add the yogurt and combine.

Apply a thin layer under and around your eyes, avoiding your eyelids.

Let it sit for 15 minutes before rinsing with cool water.

"I put frozen cucumbers on my eyes when I'm taking a bath!"
—**Noureen DeWulf, actress**

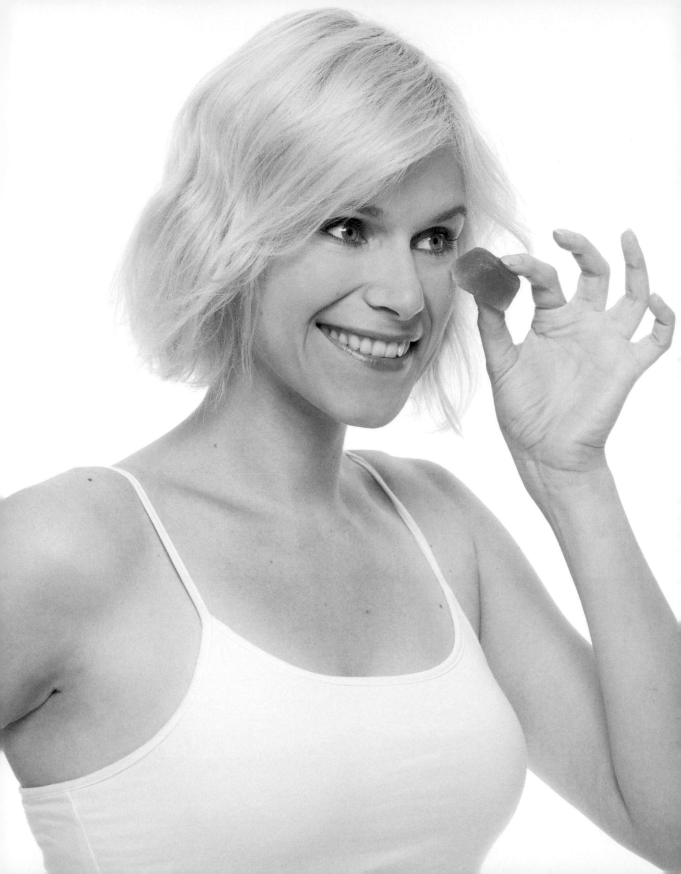

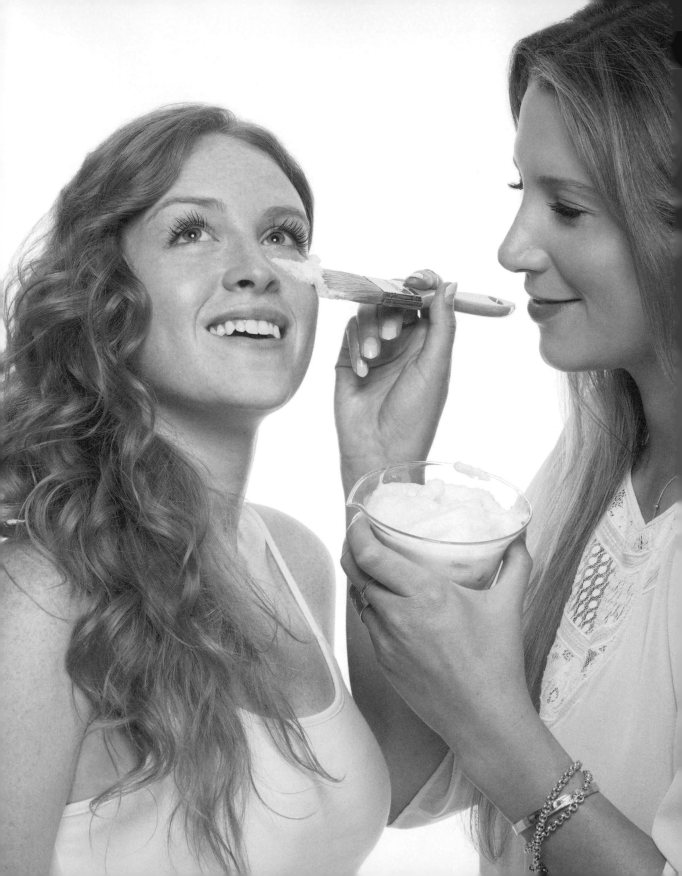

Gooseberry
Meringue Mask

All skin types

With riboflavin, a vitamin associated with improved circulation, the egg white base of this remedy helps increase blood flow to the area around your eyes, helping to de-puff and tighten. Combined with Indian gooseberry juice (also called amla juice), the richest natural source of vitamin C and a popular ayurvedic herbal drink with extraordinarily powerful anti-inflammatory properties, this eye mask will relieve swelling, redness, inflammation, and discomfort in no time.

2 egg whites

2 tablespoons Indian
   gooseberry juice (available
   at Indian grocery stores
   and many health food stores)

Using a hand blender, beat the egg whites until stiff and able to hold their form.

Slowly fold in gooseberry juice.

Apply to your eye area using a pastry brush or your fingers.

Let it sit for 15 minutes before rinsing with tepid water.

Quick Tips

• Chill out! Just like an ice pack helps assuage swollen limbs, anything cool will help to reduce redness and swelling around your eyes, too. Try frozen peas in Ziplock bags or metal spoons dipped in ice water.

• Iced coffee does more than perk up your energy! To reduce eye redness, dip cotton pads in iced black coffee and apply over closed lids for 10 minutes.

• Sleep with your head slightly elevated to reduce the amount of fluid that accumulates underneath your eyes.

• Tight on time? Apply an eye cream with caffeine listed on the packaging as an active ingredient. It constricts blood vessels to diminish discoloration and reduce puffiness. For an added bonus, keep it in the refrigerator so the chill can simultaneously work to ease your under eye woes!

"When girls show up with red eyes, I steep an organic chamomile tea bag and an organic green tea bag in a few inches of hot water for 5 minutes. I take the bags out, add ice to chill the liquid, and dip two thick cotton pads in. Place over the eyes for 3 minutes and voilà! Chamomile soothes the skin while caffeine from the green tea reduces puffiness and constricts blood vessels to take down the redness quickly."

   —Katey Denno, celebrity makeup artist

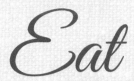

Eat

Food Cures for Red, Itchy, Puffy, Bloodshot Eyes

Ready to invest in a lifetime supply of Visine because your eyes are so red, itchy, puffy, and bloodshot? Look like you have a chronic case of pink eye or, even worse, worried your boss may think you're a stoner? Before you commit to dousing your eyes with drops designed to constrict the blood vessels and conceal the symptoms of your irritated irises, let's instead get to the cause of the problem and EAT our way to a solution.

If your eyes are dry, bloodshot, itchy, or swollen, there are all-natural solutions conveniently located in your kitchen. Did you know that lutein in broccoli protects eyes, asparagus has redness-reducing riboflavin, fish prevents dryness, and honey fights allergies? Read on for the recipes you need to clear your eyes and free them from discomfort and discoloration, from the inside out.

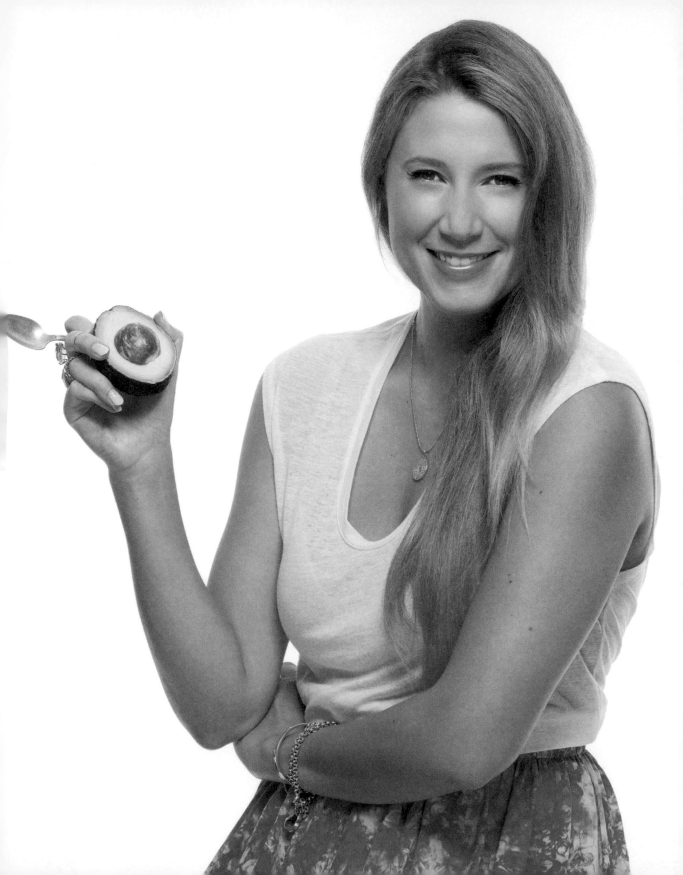

Cereal Crusted Asparagus Fries +
Yogurt Dipping Sauce

Vegetarian

If you chronically suffer with bloodshot eyes (and a lack of sleep isn't to blame!), it's possible that a riboflavin deficiency could be the culprit. Asparagus, fortified cereals, and milk are all great sources—and with such a delicious riboflavin-rich dish at hand, why not try it for the sake of your eyes?

Serves 4

YOGURT DIPPING SAUCE

1 cup fat-free Greek yogurt

1 clove garlic, minced

1 tablespoon chopped fresh dill

1 teaspoon lemon zest

1 teaspoon lemon juice

½ teaspoon salt

¼ teaspoon black pepper

CEREAL CRUSTED ASPARAGUS FRIES

1 pound asparagus

½ cup sliced raw almonds

½ cup panko breadcrumbs

½ cup Special K® breakfast cereal

2 eggs

1 tablespoon whole milk

¾ cups all-purpose flour

Cooking spray

For the Yogurt Dipping Sauce

In a small bowl, combine all of the ingredients.

Cover and refrigerate for at least 90 minutes before serving.

For the Cereal Crusted Asparagus Fries

Preheat the oven to 400°F.

Wash, trim, and pat-dry the asparagus.

Combine the almonds, bread crumbs, and cereal in a food processor.

Transfer the breading mixture to a large plate.

In a small bowl, scramble the eggs and milk together.

Toss the asparagus spears in the flour before dipping in the eggs and milk. Coat with breading mixture.

Place on a parchment-lined baking sheet and lightly spray with cooking spray.

Bake for 15 minutes, or until slightly browned and crispy.

Quick Tip
• Marmite or Vegemite, a yeast spread popular in the United Kingdom and Australia, is high in riboflavin, which can help heal bloodshot eyes. Try it on toast!

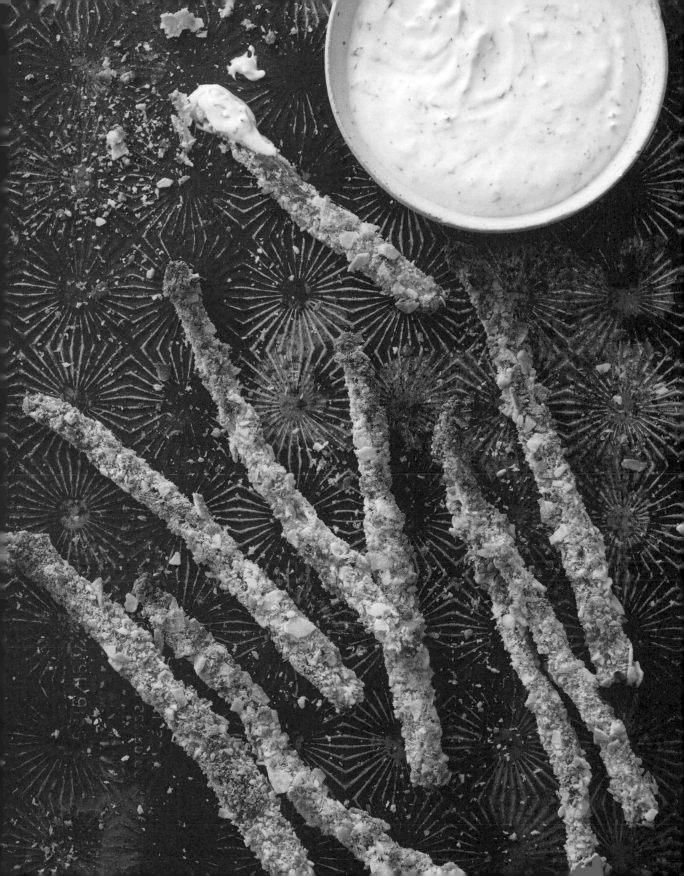

Honey Glazed Tofu + Orange Broccoli

Vegetarian, vegan, dairy-free, gluten-free, nut-free

When it comes to protecting your eyes, lutein is your knight in shining armor. Like internal sunglasses, lutein filters light to protect your eyes from sun damage and keep them healthy, sparkling, and white. Since the body doesn't produce lutein on its own, the only way to get it is through our diet. This recipe contains orange juice and broccoli, both of which boast high concentrations of eye-saving lutein. And for all you allergy sufferers, this recipe also calls for local honey, which has been shown to help stave away seasonal allergies. Bottom line: this vegan dish packs a peeper-protecting punch, while satisfying your craving for (usually unhealthy) Chinese food, too.

Serves 2

HONEY GLAZED TOFU

- 1 package (14 ounces) extra-firm water-packed tofu, drained
- ¼ cup + 2 tablespoons local honey, divided
- 3 tablespoons freshly squeezed orange juice, divided
- 1 tablespoon soy sauce
- ½ teaspoon sesame seeds
- ¼ teaspoon red pepper flakes
- 2 tablespoons extra-virgin olive oil
- ½ teaspoon salt

ORANGE BROCCOLI

- 2 cloves garlic, minced
- ⅛ teaspoon red pepper flakes
- 1 orange, zested
- 1 tablespoon extra-virgin olive oil
- ¼ cup freshly squeezed orange juice
- 1 head broccoli, cut into bite-size pieces

For the Honey Glazed Tofu

Drain and pat dry tofu before cutting into ½-inch slices.

In a shallow bowl, combine 2 tablespoons of the honey, 2 tablespoons of the orange juice, soy sauce, sesame seeds, and red pepper flakes.

Marinate the tofu in the mixture for at least 30 minutes.

In a large skillet, heat the oil, salt, and remaining honey and orange juice over medium-high heat until bubbling. Add tofu and its marinade to the skillet. Cook for 3 minutes on each side, constantly spooning sauce over tofu.

For the Orange Broccoli

In a medium saucepan, sauté the garlic, red pepper flakes, and orange zest in the oil over medium heat until the garlic is lightly browned, about 2 minutes. Add the orange juice and bring to a boil. Add the broccoli.

Cover and cook until broccoli is fork tender, about 3 minutes. Transfer to a serving dish and top with the tofu.

Quick Tip

- Sweeten food with local honey to keep allergy-induced redness away. According to Dr. Frank Lipman, integrative and functional medicine expert and founder of Eleven-Eleven Wellness Center in New York City, eating local honey can help assuage all allergy symptoms—including the eye-affecting type.

Mexicali Rockfish Ceviche

Dairy-free, gluten-free, nut-free

If your eyes are dry or inflamed, try adding more fish to your diet. Rich in omega-3 fatty acids (which most Americans are deficient in), fish helps to reduce inflammation and increase eye lubrication. Plus, rockfish contains both niacin (vitamin B3) and vitamin B12, both of which are important for helping the body to use fat and protein for healthy skin, hair, and yes, eyes. Incorporating lycopene-rich tomatoes for their antioxidant properties and hydrating avocado, this delicious ceviche will help to prevent the dryness and inflammation behind your red, irritated eyes.

Serves 2

¾ **pound rockfish fillet, deboned and thinly sliced**

4 to 6 limes, juiced and divided

1 cob corn

½ **red pepper, diced**

½ **cup halved grape tomatoes**

¼ **cup chopped spring onion**

1 tablespoon chopped cilantro

1 tablespoon extra-virgin olive oil

¼ **teaspoon salt**

¼ **teaspoon ground black pepper**

½ **thinly sliced avocado**

¼ **cup roughly chopped basil**

Cut the thinly sliced rockfish into bite-size pieces. Place the rockfish in a bowl that has a lid.

Pour the juice of 4 to 6 limes over the fish, ensuring all pieces are fully submerged. Cover the bowl and refrigerate overnight, or until the fish is opaque throughout.

Cut the kernels off of the corn and place them in a bowl with the red pepper, tomatoes, onion, and cilantro. Toss with the oil, salt, and pepper, to coat.

Drain and rinse the fish, discarding the lime juice.

Add the fish to the bowl of vegetables and toss to coat. Top with avocado and sprinkle with basil prior to serving.

Quick Tip
• Consider adding a fish or flaxseed-oil supplement to your diet. The omega-3 fatty acids help to reduce inflammation and prevent eye dryness.

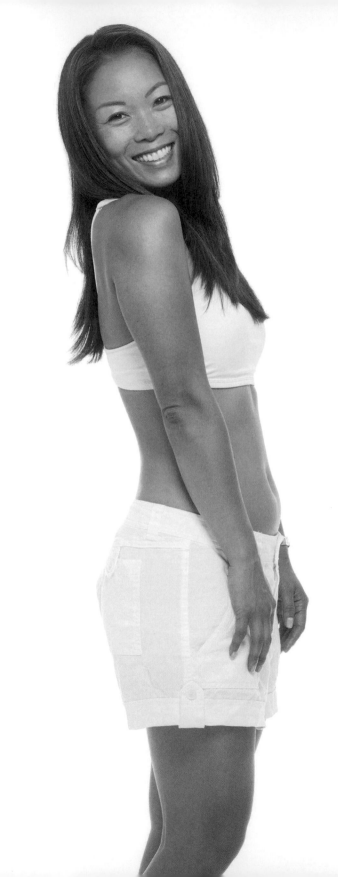

chapter 3

Body

Sunburn

Yeah, yeah, you've learned your lesson, it won't happen again . . . until it does. Perhaps you find yourself on a boat without adequate sun-protecting supplies and land far from sight; in a pool with your face precariously perched above the water (where the sun's rays bounce right off the reflective water's surface and back at your exposed face); or enjoying a cocktail at dusk unaware of the power of the sun's rays as it sets because you don't feel them; and, lo and behold, you look like a sun-dried tomato. And you feel about as cool as one, too, which is to say: not at all.

While prevention is the best medicine, sometimes that cat-nap in the sunshine still gets the best of us and we end up regrettably red and painfully peeling. Whether you're in need of immediate relief from the discomfort, hoping to stop unsightly peeling, or want to prevent the enduring effects of too much sun (like age spots, wrinkles, and even acne), you've come to the right place.

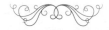

Apply

DIY Beauty Cures
for Sunburn

Hopefully you've learned your lesson and won't get burned (literally) again. But, in the meantime, you don't need to suffer with red, painful, peeling skin. With cooling compresses, soothing serums, moisturizing masks, and more, you can throw your body's natural healing processes into overdrive—stat!

Sweet Watermelon Serum

All skin types

Watermelon isn't merely a favorite summertime snack! As both a water- and vitamin-dense fruit, it also helps to moisturize, repair, and protect your skin when applied topically. Combined with honey, a natural humectant that helps pull watermelon's moisture-boosting properties deep into your skin, this serum will saturate your skin with hydrating and healing properties that will both help to prevent long-term sun damage and alleviate the immediate discomfort of sunburn. And you only need a bit of this sweet summer juice to do the trick, so you can enjoy the rest!

1 tablespoon fresh watermelon juice
1 tablespoon raw honey

Mix watermelon juice (the run-off after you slice the fruit will work) with honey until well combined.

Apply to clean, sun-kissed areas in gentle circular motions.

Let the serum penetrate for 20 minutes before rinsing residue off with cool water.

Quick Tip
• Eat a diet rich in antioxidants before sun exposure to provide added sun protection from the inside out.

Milk + Honey Calming Compresses

All skin types

Next time your skin is red and sore from too much time spent in the sun, skip the far-from-natural aloe gel and simultaneously promote healing, prevent peeling, and relieve discomfort through the power of whole milk's lactic acid and fat. Combined with the antibacterial and moisture-boosting properties of honey, these compresses will help immediately alleviate discomfort and reduce redness while also cutting healing time. Top that with antibacterial coconut oil applied to moist skin and you'll lock in healing moisture and prevent infection, too.

1 cup whole milk
3 tablespoons raw honey
1 tablespoon extra-virgin cold-pressed coconut oil

In a small bowl, mix whole milk and honey until well combined.

Saturate cotton pads (or a soft washcloth for larger areas) with the mixture and apply to sunburned skin.

As the compresses warm from your body's heat, discard and repeat until your skin is soothed.

While your skin is still moist, massage coconut oil into affected areas.

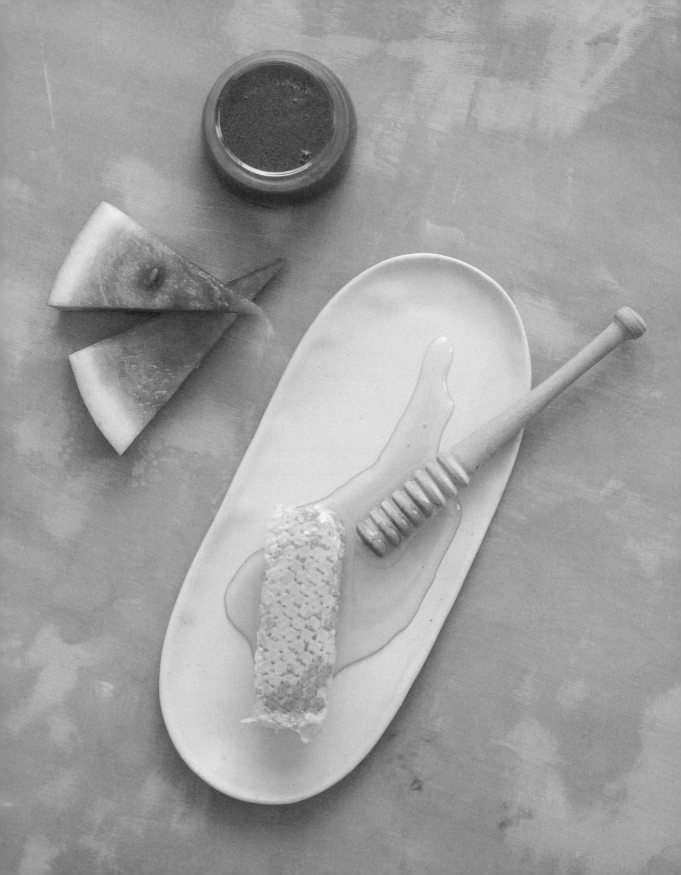

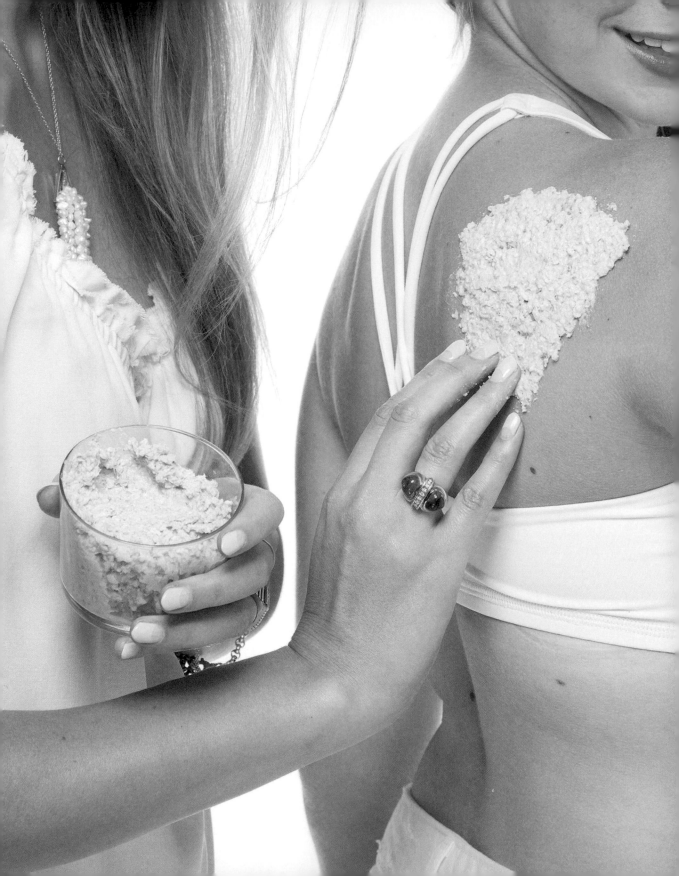

Cooling Cucumber Mask

All skin types

If your skin is currently inflamed, this calming facial mask will help to immediately soothe irritation and reduce redness. The cucumber in this recipe has antioxidants to help reverse free-radical damage, analgesic properties to assuage pain, and cooling and hydrating properties to prevent drying and peeling. Combined with anti-inflammatory oats (which work on your skin in much the same way they help to reduce your risk of heart disease), together these ingredients are a sunburn-saver. Moreover, if you're suffering from a bad reaction to a skincare product, this paste-like mask will help soothe product-induced redness and irritation as well.

1 to 2 cups oats
½ cucumber, refrigerated and peeled

In a blender, grind oatmeal until it is a flour-like consistency. Set aside.

Blend peeled cucumber until smooth. Slowly add oats to the cucumber purée, constantly stirring, until a thick paste forms. (Depending on the size of your cucumber, the amount of oats you need will vary to achieve this consistency.)

Apply a thick layer to inflamed skin for 15 minutes before rinsing with cool water.

Basil Soothing Spray

All skin types

Basil may not be the most popular of perfume scents, but if you're anything like me, you'll come to love the earthy, fresh scent of this skin-healing herb—if for no other reason than that it makes your red, irritated skin feel oh-so-much better! Mix it with summer's most popular skin-saver—fresh aloe juice, to relieve discomfort and reduce inflammation—and this refreshing spray is sure to become a beach-bag staple. Spritz it on throughout the day to promote healing by boosting circulation and reducing the risk of infection. Or just spray it on as a cooling summertime pick-me-up, whether you're sunburned or not!

3 cups water
¼ cup chopped basil leaves
4 tablespoons fresh aloe juice

Bring water to a boil before steeping basil leaves and reducing heat to a simmer, uncovered, for 15 minutes.

Remove from heat and let cool to room temperature. Stir in aloe juice and refrigerate.

Once chilled, transfer to a spray bottle and apply as needed to sun-burned skin.

Quick Tip
• Consider taking an Ibuprofen to alleviate some of the pain and reduce inflammation.

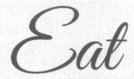

Eat

Food Cures for Sunburn

Post sunburn, your immediate concern may be aesthetic, but it's also important to encourage your body to heal itself in order to eliminate the immediate concerns (namely red, itchy, throbbing, peeling, ruddy skin) as well as the long-term consequences (namely hyperpigmentation, wrinkles, acne, and even skin cancer). With these recipes, you'll help bolster your skin's defense mechanisms to help heal sun damage more quickly than your body typically could on its own—and deliciously, too!

Shaved Fennel + Blood Orange Salad

Vegetarian, vegan, dairy-free, gluten-free, nut-free

This salad is just what your sun-damaged skin needs to heal itself from the inside out. A single cup of fennel has almost 20 percent of your recommended daily value of vitamin C, which is essential for the production and repair of collagen. Pears contain copper, an anti-inflammatory trace mineral, and blood orange has anthocyanins, which are antioxidants that fight free-radical damage and UV rays. All combined, this is just what your sunburned skin is craving.

Serves 2

1 large fennel bulb

1 Bartlett pear

2 tablespoons extra-virgin olive oil

½ lime, juiced

2 tablespoons diced fresh mint

Pinch of sea salt

1 blood orange, peeled and sectioned

Thinly slice both the fennel bulb and the pear using a mandolin slicer. Toss with the oil, lime juice, mint, and salt.

Top with the blood orange sections.

Balsamic + Goat Cheese Stuffed Figs

From Cheryl Sternman Rule, author of *Ripe: A Fresh, Colorful Approach to Fruits and Vegetables*

Vegetarian, gluten-free

Too much time spent in the sun doesn't "just" leave you uncomfortable (and less attractive!) for a few days; it also has long-term effects on your skin's aging processes. Packed with vitamin A, which is essential for glowing skin, as well as vitamin C, an antioxidant that can help fight the effects of aging, fresh figs counter the sun-induced issues that put a wrinkle in your beauty. This prettifying fig recipe is the perfect post-sun snack, and makes a great passed hors d'oeuvre at your next summertime soiree.

Serves 4 to 6

12 fresh figs, halved

4 tablespoons creamy goat cheese (plain or with black pepper)

2 tablespoons finely chopped, toasted pistachios

Cracked black pepper, to taste

Honey, to taste

High-quality balsamic vinegar, to taste

Arrange the fig halves on a platter, seed-side up.

Press ½ teaspoon of the goat cheese in the center of each fig half.

Sprinkle generously with pistachios and black pepper. Drizzle with honey and vinegar, as desired, and serve immediately.

Roasted Watermelon Gazpacho

Vegetarian, vegan, dairy-free, gluten-free, nut-free

Lycopene, found in cooked tomatoes and watermelon, helps defend against sun damage—and might even help both prevent and treat skin cancer, according to the American Cancer Society. Keep this gazpacho in your refrigerator all summer long for a skin-healing soup that's as refreshing as it is healing.

Serves 2 to 4

3 vine tomatoes, chopped

1 tablespoon extra-virgin olive oil

3 cups watermelon, seeded

1 clove garlic

2 tablespoons fresh lime juice

¼ cup roasted almonds

½ tablespoon sweet smoked paprika

1 medium cucumber, peeled and divided

Salt, to taste

Cayenne pepper (optional)

2 tablespoons diced sweet onion

On medium heat, sauté tomatoes in the oil until fork-tender. Transfer to a blender.

Add watermelon, garlic, lime juice, almonds, paprika, and half of the cucumber. Blend until smooth. Add salt to taste and cayenne pepper, if desired.

Refrigerate until chilled and ready to serve.

Stir in the diced onion.

Thinly slice the remaining cucumber.

Top the soup with the cucumber slices.

Quick Tip
• Snack on antioxidant bursting blackberries, blueberries, raspberries, and strawberries for an SPF boost from the inside out!

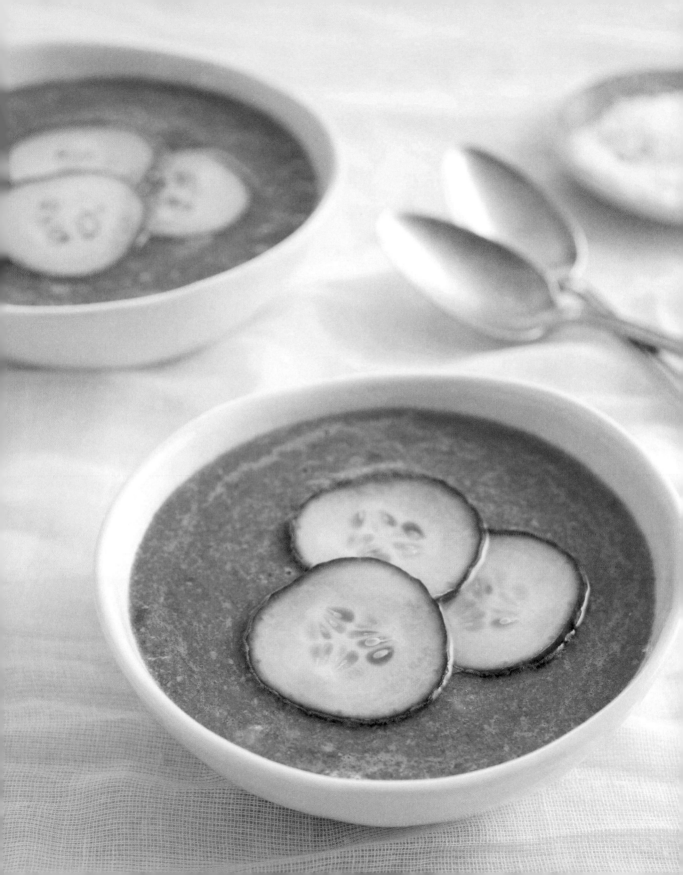

Roasted Broccoli + Sun-Dried Tomato Spaghetti

From Phoebe Lapine, FeedMePhoebe.com

Vegetarian, nut-free

With lycopene-rich sun-dried tomatoes to help protect skin from the damaging effects of too much sun, and selenium-rich whole-wheat pasta to promote elasticity, this antioxidant-rich pasta dish will help to reverse and heal past sun damage as well as keep your skin shielded from further damage. Keep leftovers in the refrigerator for a refreshing pasta salad the next day.

Serves 4

1 pound broccoli

1 tablespoon extra-virgin olive oil

½ teaspoon sea salt

1 pound whole wheat spaghetti

1 jar (10 ounces) sun-dried tomatoes in olive oil

½ teaspoon crushed red chili flakes

2 teaspoons red wine vinegar

¼ cup grated pecorino cheese, to garnish

Preheat the oven to 400°F.

Trim the broccoli into small florets.

On a parchment-lined baking sheet, toss the broccoli together with the oil and salt. Arrange in an even layer and roast in the oven until browned and caramelized, about 20 minutes.

Bring a large pot of salted water to boil. Cook the spaghetti according to package directions. Drain and set aside.

Add the sun-dried tomatoes and their oil, along with the chili flakes and vinegar, to a small food processor or blender. Purée until smooth, adding more olive oil, if necessary, until the paste resembles the texture of a thick pesto. Add more salt as necessary, to taste.

Toss the cooked pasta and roasted broccoli with the tomato paste.

Divide between 4 bowls and garnish with pecorino.

Quick Tip

• Studies have shown that regularly eating omega-3 fatty acids increases the skin's immunity to sunlight. Add a sprinkle of chia seeds to your next smoothie recipe for a skin-protecting boost!

Classic Collard Greens

From Wendy Williams, TV host

Dairy-free, gluten-free, nut-free

When Wendy Williams isn't on the set of her daytime talk show, *The Wendy Williams Show*, the host is all about wiping off the TV makeup and letting her true self shine. I met her backstage, just minutes after taping her show. Immediately the makeup came off and her gorgeous glow shown through. Naturally, I asked her to share her best recipe for beauty! While Wendy makes her collard greens for their powerful and widespread beauty benefits, I particularly love collards for their skin-saving effects. Packed with vitamin E to encourage healing, vitamin K to optimize circulation, and calcium to help your skin stay hydrated, Wendy's collard greens recipe is perfect post-sun fare.

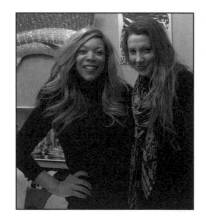

Serves 4

1 ham hock

2 cloves garlic

Hot sauce, to taste

1 pound collard greens, roughly chopped

¼ teaspoon salt

¼ teaspoon black pepper

Sauté the ham hock, garlic, and hot sauce in about 3 inches of water over low-medium heat for about 30 to 45 minutes, covered.

Once the ham hock is tender, add the collard greens. Make sure the greens are at least halfway covered with water, adding more if needed. Season with the salt and pepper, cover, and reduce to a low heat for about 2 hours.

Remove from heat but keep covered for another hour, allowing the greens to marinate.

Add more salt, pepper, garlic, and hot sauce, as desired to taste.

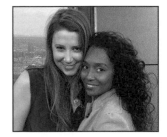

Quick Tip

• Don't drain any remaining liquid from your collards. Instead slurp it up! TLC's Chilli (who, for the record, doesn't seem to have aged one bit from the 1994 cover of *CrazySexyCool*) told me that when she sautés kale and collards, she drinks the remaining water like a soup or serves it with cooked whole lentils. "That's where all the nutrients are!"

Cellulite

Unless we're looking at a picture and there is Photoshop involved, you likely have cellulite. We all do. Or at least an estimated 85–90 percent of us! Sure, working your butt off at the gym helps, as does having the genetic makeup of a swimsuit model, but the fact is, sometimes even that isn't enough. Have you seen the cover of those trashy magazines by the checkout line of the grocery store lately? Even women who pay loads of money to look "flawless" have some cellulite. Luckily, you probably don't have paparazzi following you around, pining for a picture of your unwanted dimples!

Unlike other forms of fat storage on our bodies, cellulite isn't necessarily indicative of having too much fat on your body (phew!). In fact, lots of super-skinny girls have it! Cellulite is what you see when your skin's elastic fibers that hold everything in place deteriorate to the point that the fat cells push through your skin's dermis layer, becoming visible right below the uppermost layer of skin. Jealous your main man doesn't seem to have any cellulite? Well, it's not necessarily because he's in better shape than you are. Genetically, men tend to have more—and stronger—connective tissue under the surface of the skin, holding their fat layer deep below.

Assuming you like your cottage cheese with a spoon, not on your thighs, you can rest assured: the appearance of cellulite isn't inevitable. Yes, even with the vast majority of women suffering with it, there are still things we can do. Namely, we can EAT to bolster our collagen production, which is responsible for keeping fat cells well beneath the skin's visible surface, and we can APPLY to temporarily conceal the appearance of cellulite until our bodies are able to keep it in place all by itself.

Here's how . . .

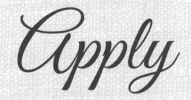

DIY Beauty Cures
for Cellulite

Dimpled thighs got you down? Stop hiding under layers of skin-covering clothes and pull out that string bikini (come on, I know you have at least one somewhere!) because your dimpled skin is about to be baby-bottom smooth. With caffeine, manual exfoliation, and massage to bring blood flow to the surface of the skin, you can temporarily conceal the appearance of cellulite before a day at the beach or night out in a shorter-than-usual skirt.

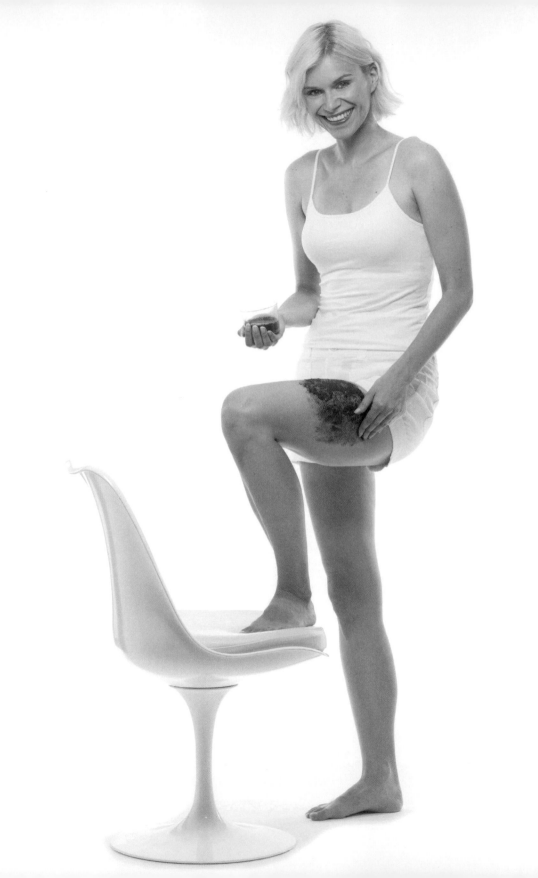

Cellulite-Concealing Coffee Scrub

All skin types

Look at the package on the most expensive cellulite creams on the market and the one ingredient you're bound to see appear over and over again is caffeine. Because of its ability to temporarily increase blood flow at the skin's surface (which plumps up the dimples) as well as flush out the water in the connective tissue (which deflates the lumps), caffeine is highly effective at making devilish dimples disappear.

There's no need to spend lots of money on an ingredient you can get (very cheaply!) in your own kitchen. Mixed with wheat germ oil, which is rich in skin-saving vitamin E to help skin heal itself from the inside out, this coffee scrub is bound to become one of your favorite beach-ready remedies. Plus, this cellulite-concealing scrub is chemical-free, so you don't need to worry about all those other ingredients you can't pronounce on the store-bought solutions.

½ cup caffeinated coffee grounds

¼ cup wheat germ oil

Mix the coffee grounds and wheat germ oil together to form a thick paste.

Standing in the bath to reduce mess, apply the mixture to cellulite-covered skin.

Cover it with tightly wrapped plastic wrap and let it sit for 30 minutes.

Remove wrap before vigorously rubbing the mixture in upward circular motions for at least 5 minutes.

Rinse clean with warm water.

Since the results of this scrub are temporary, for best results repeat daily.

Note: You can use either fresh or used (but cooled!) coffee grounds in this recipe.

Quick Tip
- Self-tanner—or even bronzer—can help conceal the appearance of cellulite. It's a trick models and celebrities like Kim Kardashian swear by. The shimmer distracts and conceals for more flawless-looking legs.

Detoxifying Seaweed Bath

All skin types

You may think you need to be working your butt off to, well, work your butt off, but the fact is you can soak your cellulite away in a relaxing bath. With seaweed to promote circulation, whole milk to gently exfoliate and moisturize, honey to hydrate, and salt to detoxify, this bath soak will take your usually boring bath to spa-like depths as it reduces the appearance of cellulite.

1 cup whole milk
¼ cup honey
1 cup dried seaweed or powdered kelp
½ cup sea salt

Combine the whole milk and honey.

Under running water, pour the milk and honey into a warm bath. Add the seaweed or kelp and salt prior to getting in the bath.

Soak for 20 to 30 minutes before rinsing off.

Note: Dried seaweed and powdered kelp are available in the international food section of most grocery stores or at any Asian market.

Coconut Polish

Not for sensitive or acne-prone skin

Dry-brushing skin has long been a tried-and-trusted solution for cellulite for a host of reasons. It stimulates the lymphatic system to detoxify, increases skin's blood flow, exfoliates and tightens skin, and encourages cell renewal, all of which work to rid the body of toxins and reduce the appearance of cellulite. Combine it with coconut oil, which hydrates, plumps, and gently exfoliates and you'll be cellulite-free in no time!

2 tablespoons extra-virgin cold-pressed coconut oil
Dry brush, natural bristles

Massage affected areas with the coconut oil for 5 minutes before using a dry brush with natural bristles to gently but vigorously brush cellulite, using long sweeps in the direction of your heart. If you're brushing your stomach, brush counter-clockwise.

Skin should be invigorated, not irritated.

Quick Tip
• Strong muscles make cellulite less obvious. Do some squats while watching TV to keep legs lean and taut!

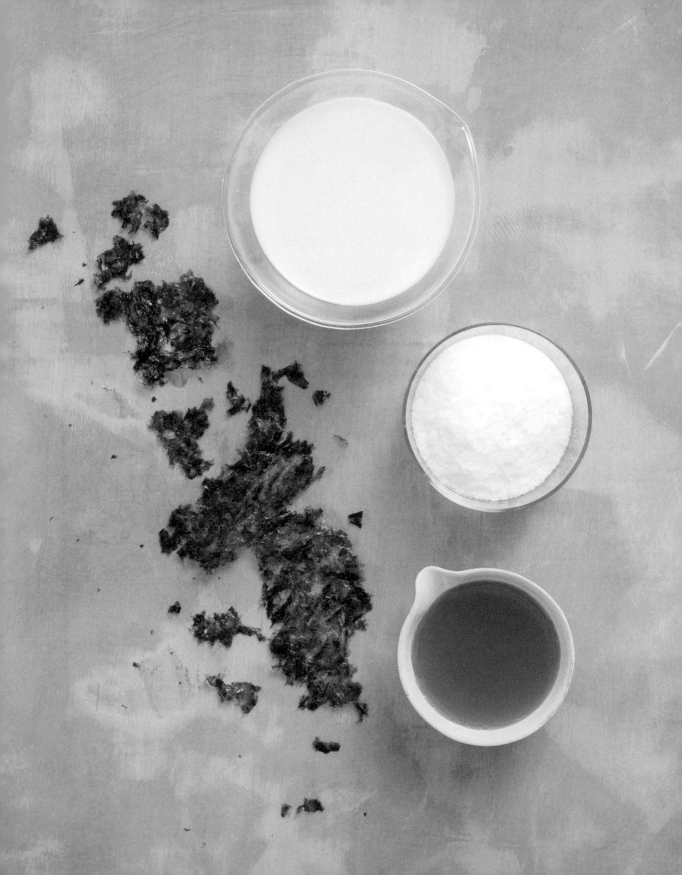

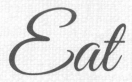

Eat

Food Cures for Cellulite

You may think that an anti-cellulite diet means a fat-free one, but the same way having a lot of cellulite isn't indicative of having a large percentage of body fat, eating fat is unrelated to the appearance of cellulite. So what is the key to an anti-cellulite diet? Together, more collagen, stronger elastin, and increased circulation ensure your fat cells stay held securely beneath the skin's surface and don't peek out in their dimple-like way (which sounds way cuter than it is!). Also, increasing your metabolism helps by keeping additional fat deposits away—because, of course, if there's no fat there to peek out, there can be no cellulite in the first place!

Raw Creamsicle Milk Shake

Vegetarian, vegan, dairy-free, gluten-free, nut-free

Tropical and citrus fruits, like pineapples, papayas, and oranges, are all high in vitamin C, which helps your body produce collagen, a protein that helps your skin maintain its firmness and elasticity from the inside out. Plus, bioflavonoids, found in citrus fruits, help strengthen capillaries and increase circulation, both of which can help your body to flush away cellulite—or at the very least, help to make it less obvious. Add raw coconut meat, which is not only deliciously creamy but also high in medium-chain fatty acids, which studies show may boost your metabolism, and this milk shake will help make you look better at your next pool party!

Serves 1 to 2

1 large naval orange, peeled and frozen

¼ cup pineapple cubes, fresh or frozen

¼ cup papaya cubes, fresh or frozen

1 ½ cups raw coconut meat (or the meat from 2 young Thai coconuts)

½ to 1 cup coconut water, as desired

Peel and freeze the naval orange overnight, or longer.

In a blender, combine fruit and coconut meat and begin to blend. Slowly add coconut water until all ingredients are combined and you achieve desired consistency.

Note: I always buy oranges in bulk, but after I know I won't use them when fresh, I peel and freeze them to make this milk shake!

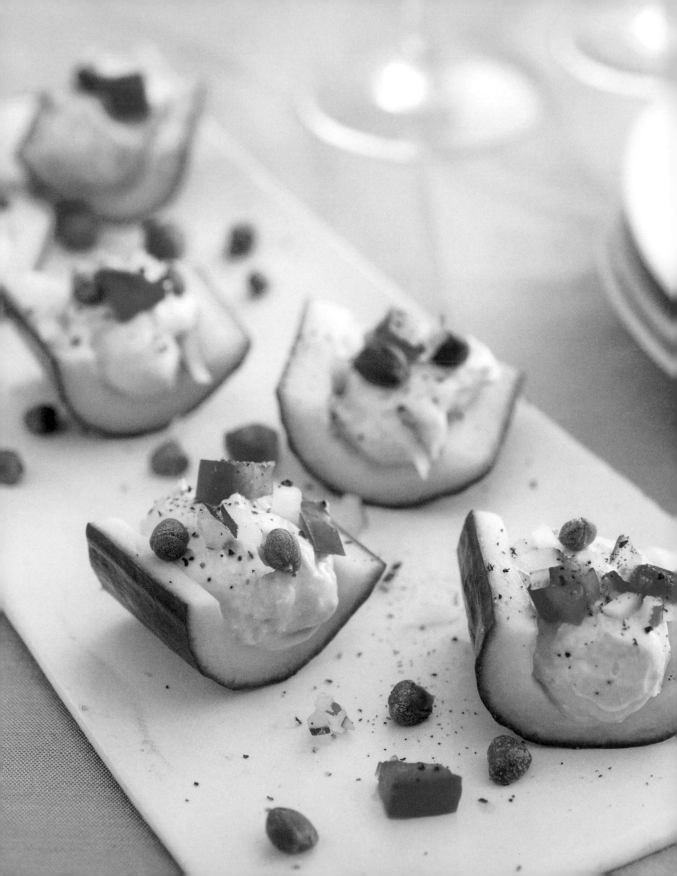

Creamy Salmon Cucumber Boats

Gluten-free, nut-free

Next time you're looking for an easy hors d'oeuvre to serve at a dinner party, or just a quick but seemingly decadent lunch idea, try these fresh cucumber boats. They're protein-packed with cottage cheese and salmon to support strong muscles, which are essential in appearing cellulite-free, and cucumber skin boasts an impressive amount of silica, which boosts collagen production. On top of that, these "boats" taste like a bagel with lox, and who doesn't love a healthy take on an indulgent brunch staple?

Serves 6

½ cup low-fat cottage cheese, drained

¼ cup whipped cream cheese

1 tablespoon low-fat or skim milk

4 ounces smoked salmon

1 tablespoon fresh lemon juice

½ teaspoon fresh ground white pepper

2 12-inch cucumbers

½ vine tomato, seeded and diced

1 tablespoon capers

1 tablespoon diced purple onion

In a food processor, combine the cottage cheese, cream cheese, and milk until smooth. Add the salmon, lemon, and pepper and process until creamy.

Transfer to a bowl, cover, and refrigerate for 1 hour.

Cut the cucumbers once in half, lengthwise, and then in thirds to create twelve 4-inch pieces. Use a spoon to scoop out the seeds and discard.

Evenly divide the creamy salmon filling among the "boats."

Sprinkle with diced tomatoes, capers, and onion. Top with additional ground pepper and lemon, if desired.

Chopped Veggie Spice Salad

Tara Stiles, model turned yoga guru

Vegetarian, vegan, dairy-free, gluten-free, nut-free

Tara Stiles is one of the few women I'm confident is actually cellulite-free, even (for the record!) without having seen her naked. So after the superstar yogi told me that this chopped vegetable salad recipe is one of her favorite beauty-boosting recipes, I booked it to the grocery store to whip it up. Like Spanx in a bowl, this salad, with all of its colorful vegetables, effectively supports collagen production, sucking things in and preventing lumps and bumps from peeking out. Up the ante in this recipe by adding hot sauce, which helps boost your metabolism.

Serves 1 to 2

Handful of chopped kale (about 1 cup)

Handful of baby spinach (about 1 cup)

1 celery stalk

1 carrot

½ cucumber

½ red bell pepper

½ lemon

1 tablespoon balsamic vinegar

¼ tablespoon Dijon mustard

¼ teaspoon hot sauce

Chop all of the kale, baby spinach, celery, carrot, cucumber, and red bell pepper into bite-size pieces and combine in a mixing bowl.

Squeeze the lemon over the vegetables and massage with hands until the kale is tender.

In a small bowl, combine vinegar, Dijon mustard, and hot sauce, stirring until smooth. Pour over vegetables and serve immediately.

Quick Tip
- Water is to cellulite as kryptonite is to Superman: deadly. Chug H_2O or munch on water-rich fruits and veggies, like watermelon, to flush away bloat and reduce the appearance of cellulite.

Mediterranean Turkey Burgers

From Danielle Rehfeld, chef

Dairy-free, nut-free

Want to rock that cellulite-free, dimple-free body of yours all summer long? Steer clear of the usual poolside hamburger and instead throw a turkey burger on the grill! With its high concentration of zinc, turkey helps to support your body's collagen and elastin fibers, which together work to preserve and promote skin's elasticity and firmness from the inside out.

Serves 4

2 pounds ground white meat turkey

1 small yellow onion, grated (about ½ cup)

2 cups cilantro leaves, chopped

2 cups parsley leaves, chopped

3 cloves garlic, minced

1 egg

½ cup dry seasoned bread crumbs

1 ½ teaspoons kosher salt

¾ teaspoons freshly ground black pepper

¾ teaspoon Aleppo pepper

¼ teaspoon turmeric powder

¼ teaspoon ground cumin

Pinch of ground cinnamon

Canola oil, for brushing

Place all of the ingredients in a large bowl and mix well.

Form 4 patties. Cover tightly with plastic wrap and refrigerate for at least 1 hour or up to 24 hours before grilling.

Heat a large nonstick pan or stovetop grill over medium-high heat. Brush lightly with oil.

When the oil begins to shimmer, season the patties with a little salt and grill for 5 minutes on the first side.

Flip and cook for 5 minutes on the second side, covering for the last 1 ½ minutes of cooking. Rest 1 to 2 minutes.

Serve with finely chopped cilantro, jalapeño, lemon juice, and salt, if desired.

Note: As a make-ahead meal, wrap these burgers individually in plastic wrap and store them in the freezer. Defrost in the refrigerator 24 hours prior to cooking.

Body Breakouts

When it comes to confidently rocking an open back or showing off your shoulders in a tank top, little gets in the way more than a bad case of bacne (or shoulder-cne, although that doesn't slip off the tongue nearly as well). Worse of all, oftentimes body breakouts occur just as the weather warms and the sunshine seems to be begging us to strip off our layers and show off our skin!

Hair product residue may be clogging your pores. Hormones could be causing breakouts. Your not-nearly-as-exfoliated-as-necessary skin may be speckled with white or red bumps. For a lot of different reasons, body breakouts can happen to the best of us. Even those of us with relatively clear complexions sometimes find ourselves self-consciously concealing a blemish on our back, chest, shoulder, or even butt.

Before you banish backless from your vocabulary and ditch all the body-baring clothes in your closet, let's tackle those body breakouts once and for all, in your kitchen no less. With an anti-inflammatory and skin-clearing diet combined with a pore-clearing, redness-reducing, and exfoliating skincare regimen, your skin can be clear, smooth, and bump-free—and you'll be able to show it confidently.

Apply

DIY Beauty Cures
for Body Breakouts

The more-delicate APPLY recipes from Chapter 1 of this book that fight the pimples wreaking havoc on your face will work on your body as well (so feel free to whip up larger batches of those recipes and use them on your body as well!), but when it comes to waging war on body breakouts, you can pull out the big guns. Where your facial skin is sensitive to the effects of harsh products, your body can usually take a little extra. Just remember: the reverse isn't true and the recipes here are too strong for the more sensitive skin on your face, neck, and décolleté.

Yogurt + Baking Soda Buffer

All skin types

Full-fat Greek yogurt is one of the best kept blemish busting secrets. With lactic acid to gently exfoliate, probiotics to balance good and bad bacteria, and fat to moisturize without clogging pores, it's one of the easiest and most effective ways to instantly reduce inflammation and redness. Mix in baking soda, which is slightly antiseptic, to manually buff away dead skin cells, and your acne-covered skin will not just look instantly less red, bumpy, and clogged, it will be less prone to breakouts going forward, too.

½ cup full-fat Greek yogurt
½ cup baking soda

Mix the yogurt and the baking soda until well combined.

Apply a thick layer to affected areas and let it dry for 20 minutes.

Use circular motions to scrub the majority of the mask off before rinsing the remainder off with warm water.

Follow with a splash of cold water to close your pores.

Strawberry Clearing Mask

Not for sensitive skin

With five different types of acids and a hefty dose of vitamin C, strawberries are a great way to gently break down dead skin cells, exfoliate clogged pores, and wash skin in antioxidants. Add in highly acidic lemons and antibacterial honey and this sweet-and-sour body mask is your body breakout's worst nightmare.

8 medium strawberries, destemmed
2 lemons, juiced
4 tablespoons raw honey

In a food processor, purée the strawberries and lemon juice until smooth.

Transfer to a bowl before stirring in the honey.

Apply a thick layer to affected areas and let it stand for 15 to 20 minutes.

Rinse with warm water.

Quick Tips

• Mix baking soda with water to form a paste and apply as an overnight spot treatment to kill bacteria and dry out blemishes.

• Having trouble treating hard to reach areas? Put the APPLY remedies on a spatula for easier application!

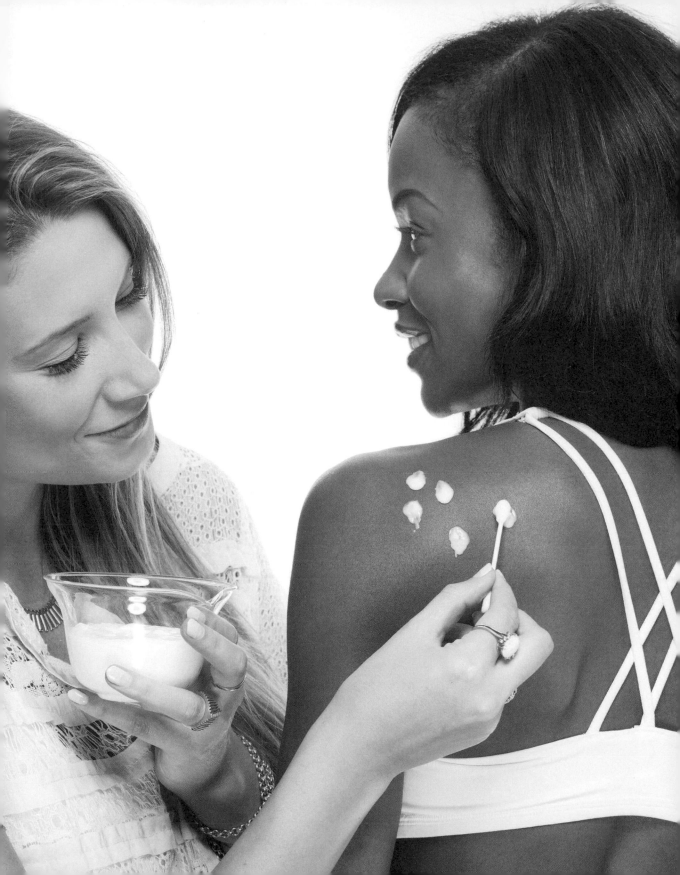

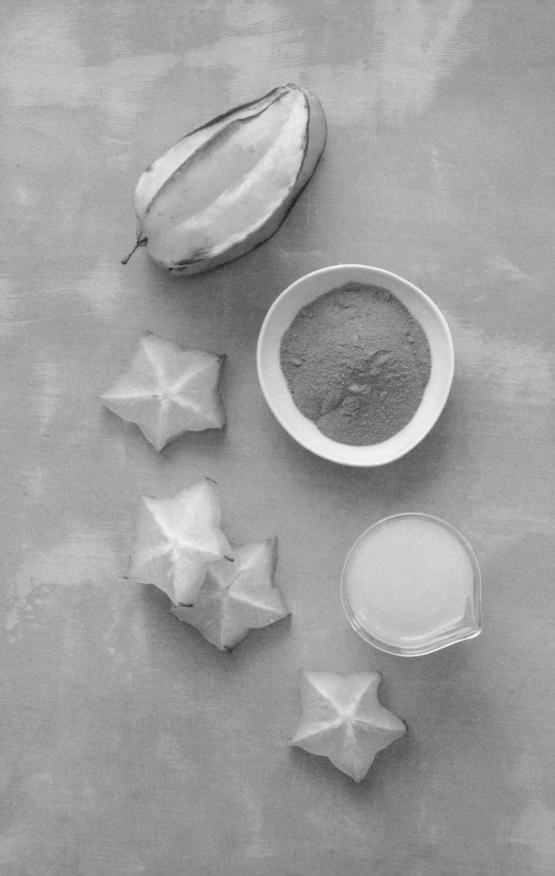

Starry Spot Treatment

All skin types

Starfruit (also called carambola) is both rich in oil-busting and exfoliating vitamin A and high in vitamin C, which protects skin against sun damage, meaning it will also help to prevent future breakouts caused by too much time in the sun. The lime juice in this treatment helps to exfoliate dead skin cells, shrink pores, and may even help kill germs when applied topically. Combined with turmeric, which has antiseptic and anti-inflammatory properties, and this spot treatment is bound to send those body breakouts into oblivion—where they belong!

1 starfruit

2 tablespoons fresh lime juice

1 teaspoon turmeric

In a food processor, purée the starfruit with the lime juice until smooth. Add the turmeric and mix until well combined.

Laying so that the affected areas are flat and the treatment doesn't slide off, apply as thick of a layer as will adhere and let it sit for 15 to 20 minutes.

Rinse with cool water.

Quick Tips

• Crush an aspirin (a pure form of salicylic acid) and mix it with 5 drops of lemon juice to spot treat a body blemish. If you feel irritation, remove immediately—and never use this on your face.

• Add a few tablespoons of white sugar to your body wash immediately before use to gently exfoliate pore-clogging dead skin cells.

• Toss your loofah, which can harbor acne-causing bacteria. Instead, use a washcloth and wash it regularly.

• Your favorite hair products could be the cause of your clogged pores! After shampooing and conditioning your hair, use a clip to keep hair product residue off your skin while cleansing your body last—and use a separate towel just for your hair to prevent transference.

"Out of the blue in my late twenties my back started breaking out! I used this trick to combat them: in a small plastic bowl add 1/2 cup old-fashioned oatmeal and mix with water to create a paste, then add 3 tablespoons ground almonds and a few drops of either grape seed or olive oil. Rub and scrub your back or full body with this mixture to remove dead skin and soothe good skin."

—Tara Loren, celebrity makeup artist

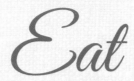

Eat

Food Cures
for Body Breakouts

As with facial breakouts, body breakouts are often caused by some combination of hormones, overactive oil production, bacteria, and dead skin cells that fail to exfoliate, instead sticking around to clog unwelcoming pores. Just as we EAT for faces free from acne, we can EAT to banish body breakouts by reducing inflammation and fostering healing to quickly eliminate existing breakouts. We'll also focus on encouraging faster cell turnover and reducing oil production to prevent future breakouts.

Pack your plate with vitamin A to help your body exfoliate from the inside out, vitamin E to promote faster healing, zinc to control oil-production, and loads of anti-inflammatories (in greens, beef, and nuts!), and your body breakouts will be a thing of the past.

Bocconcino di Tartara

From Gabriele Corcos and Debi Mazar, *Extra Virgin*, New York City

Dairy-free, gluten-free, nut-free

You may not think of beef tartar as a beauty food—but think again! High in zinc, beef (in moderation) can reduce inflammation and slow oil production, helping to both banish existing blemishes and prevent new ones from forming. This decadent, slightly-seared, French take on steak tartare steers clear of the typical accoutrements in favor of vitamin C-rich caramelized lemons, which also help to both clear and heal body breakouts from the inside out for a beauty-boosting dish meat-lovers will, well—love!

Serves 4

1 lemon, sliced ¼ inch thick

¼ pound center-cut beef fillet

Extra-virgin olive oil, as needed

1 lemon, zested

Sea salt, to taste

Preheat a griddle over high heat.

Sear the lemon slices on the griddle on each side until they become slightly caramelized. Remove from heat and set aside.

Chop the fillet as finely as possible, by hand, using a sharp knife.

Form the chopped meat into loose balls, about 2 ounces each.

Sear only the bottoms of the meatballs on the griddle with oil. Serve immediately over the grilled lemon slices. Top with lemon zest and salt.

Giardino

From Nick Anderer, executive chef/partner at Maialino, New York City

Vegetarian, vegan, dairy-free, gluten-free, nut-free

Drink for breakout-free skin with this sweet green juice recipe from chef Nick Anderer. With anti-inflammatory greens and fennel, hydrating cucumber and celery, and detoxifying fruits, this sweet sip of greens will encourage your body to flush out pore-clogging toxins and absorb anti-inflammatory vitamins for clean, glowing skin from head to toe.

Serves 2

2 Granny Smith apples

2 pears

1 large bunch of kale (about 2 cups)

1 fennel bulb

1 cucumber

2 celery stalks

Wash vegetables and fruit thoroughly.

Cut all ingredients into large chunks that fit easily in a juicer. Process cut-up vegetables and fruits in the juicer.

Enjoy immediately.

Creamy Butternut Squash Porridge

Vegetarian, vegan, dairy-free, gluten-free

Make a breakout-busting breakfast with this anti-inflammatory and skin-clearing porridge recipe. Loaded with beta-carotene—which your body converts to vitamin A—butternut squash works to ensure your cells turn over properly and remain both unclogged and radiant. Combine the butternut squash with vitamin E and riboflavin-packed almonds, which promote healing, reduce inflammation, and prevent free-radical damage and eat your way to a breakout-free body!

Serves 2 to 4

¼ cup raw walnuts

¼ cup raw almonds

1 large butternut squash, peeled and cubed

2 tablespoons extra-virgin olive oil

3 tablespoons maple syrup, divided

1 teaspoon cinnamon

1 teaspoon nutmeg

½ to 1 cup almond milk

Salt, to taste

Soak the walnuts and almonds in enough water to cover overnight.

Preheat the oven to 425°F.

Toss the cubed butternut squash with the oil and 2 tablespoons of the maple syrup before placing on a baking sheet. Roast for 30 minutes or until the squash is tender.

Drain the walnuts and almonds.

In a food processor, combine the nuts, butternut squash, cinnamon, and nutmeg. Slowly add the almond milk until you have a thick porridge.

Top with remaining maple syrup and salt, to taste.

Quick Tips

• One cup of dried watermelon seeds (popular in East Asia and the Middle East) has over 70 percent of your recommended daily value of breakout-busting zinc. Find them in Asian food markets and sprinkle them on salads for crunch.

• Oysters aren't just an aphrodisiac; they can also help you to actually look sexier by preventing acne!

• Swap your usual white bread or pasta for whole grains to keep blood sugar levels stable and acne away!

• Snack on walnuts, which have tryptophan. The stress-reducing amino acid can help prevent hormonal breakouts.

• Top your next salad with fatty fish (like salmon, albacore tuna, halibut, or sardines), which are high in inflammation-reducing omega-3 fatty acids.

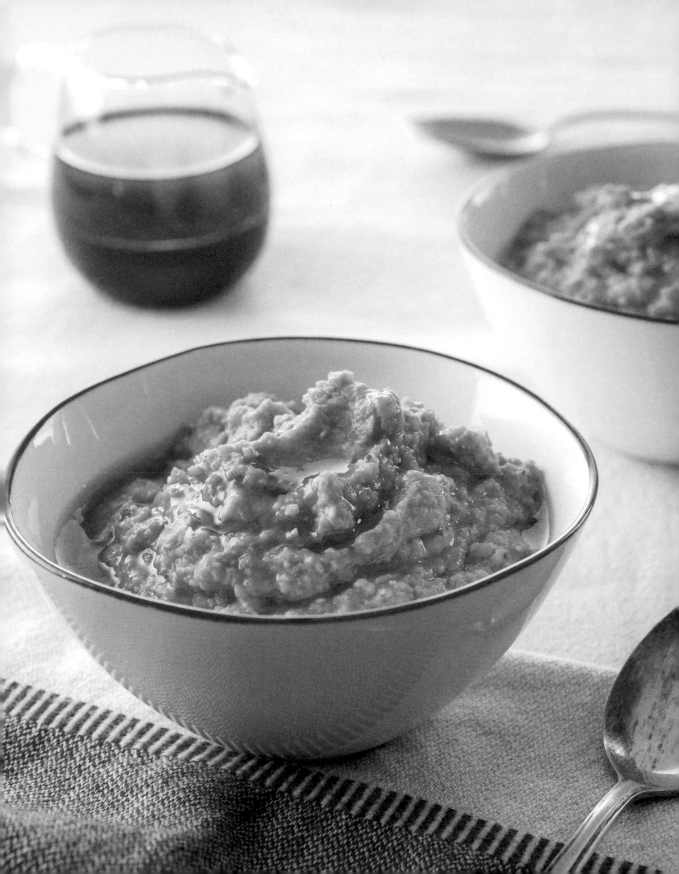

Stretch Marks

When skin is forced to stretch faster than it can grow to accommodate a larger physique the result is—you guessed it—stretch marks.

For some women, it's a puberty-induced growth spurt that leave hips and breasts with ribbons of lighter flesh. For others, it's due to hormonal changes. For me, it was recovering from an eating disorder that left me with some stretch marks on my inner thighs and bum. And as much as I would like to think of my stretch marks as a badge of honor—my current ones as a sign of a struggle overcome; future ones if I'm fortunate to have a baby one day, as a sign of my powerful body's ability to create life—let's be honest here: no matter my appreciation for where my body's been, how far it's come and how far it may go, I find stripes of purple or white announcing such, entirely unnecessary.

Before we dive into EATing and APPLYing for stretchmark-free skin, though, I want to set expectations here. Although we can APPLY and EAT our way to stretchmark-less skin by fading them and helping to prevent future ones, entirely eliminating stretch marks is something not even high-powered (and extraordinarily expensive) laser resurfacing machines can do and, alas, neither can the foods in our kitchen.

All is not lost, though; read on for beauty recipes that can help to diminish the stretch marks you currently have and hinder the onset of future ones.

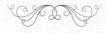

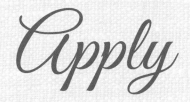

Apply

DIY Beauty Cures for Stretch Marks

Sure, there are a lot of remedies on the market that you can buy to help prevent and heal stretch marks, but many of them are loaded with chemicals that I wouldn't suggest applying them on growing girls or pregnant women (especially on a pregnant stomach). And, more often than not, even their results leave much to be desired. As a result, many women find themselves thinking of their stretch marks as nothing short of an inevitable byproduct of puberty and pregnancy.

But they're not.

Here you'll find topical remedies that will increase your skin's elasticity (to help prevent further stretch marks) and promote your skin's healing (to reduce the appearance of existing ones). And, with all-natural ingredients that you can feel good about your skin absorbing, they're safe for growing girls and pregnant women, the two groups most prone to stretch marks.

When fading stretch marks topically, keep in mind that the newer the stretch mark, the faster it will fade. So start with these APPLY remedies as soon as possible for the best results.

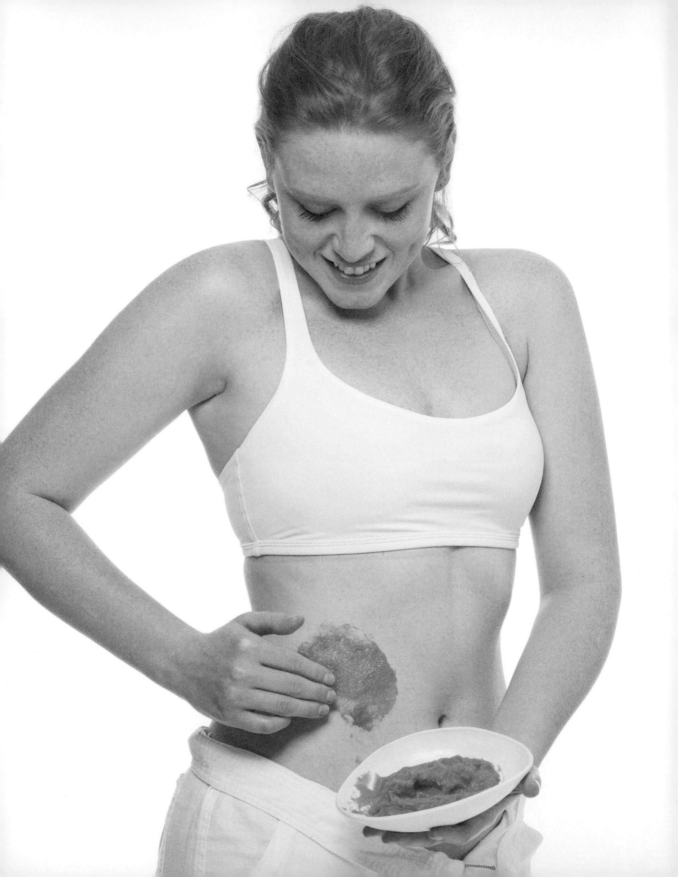

Sweet Potato + Honey Healer

All skin types

Retinols may be one of the go-to prescription treatments for healing stretch marks topically, but they cannot be applied during pregnancy. And, if they're not safe for pregnant women, you may not want to apply them to non-expectant skin either. Retinols, though, get their power from vitamin A—the same vitamin A found in sweet potatoes! In this recipe the sweet potato is combined with manuka honey, which has both antibacterial and anti-inflammatory properties and has been shown to help stimulate collagen production and the growth of new tissue. Bottom line: this sweet mask can help to effectively fade existing stretch marks—100 percent naturally!

1 medium sweet potato, peeled and chopped
¼ cup manuka honey

In a medium pot, boil the sweet potato in water until easily pierced with a fork, approximately 20 minutes.

Drain and transfer to a food processor. Add the honey and blend until smooth and well combined.

Let it cool to room temperature before applying a thick layer to stretch marks. Let it sit for 20 minutes before rinsing with warm water.

Repeat daily for best results.

Rejuvenating Scar Scrub

Not for very sensitive skin

Fading stretch marks is as much about fading surface damage as it is about promoting elasticity and collagen production deeper within the skin. Lactic, citric, and lauric acids (in milk, lemon juice, and coconut oil, respectively) work together to gently chemically exfoliate. Add a manual exfoliator—sugar—to the mix, and this scrub will help to fade stretch marks by sloughing off dead skin cells, encouraging cell turnover, and fading discoloration.

2 tablespoons whole milk
2 tablespoons lemon juice
2 tablespoons extra-virgin cold-pressed
    coconut oil
¼ cup white sugar

Combine the milk, lemon juice, and coconut oil. Stir in the sugar and immediately massage into affected areas for 5 to 7 minutes.

Rinse with warm water and follow with the Ginger + Turmeric Massage Oil (recipe on page 158).

Ginger + Turmeric
Massage Oil

All skin types

By increasing collagen production, which boosts your skin's elasticity, and reducing free-radical damage, which can interfere in your skin's natural ability to heal, vitamin E is a double-whammy stretch mark healer. Wheat germ oil is loaded with it! The other two ingredients in this recipe, ginger and turmeric, are popular in South Asia for their wound-repairing and collagen-boosting properties. Best of all for moms-to-be, because these ingredients are all-natural and food-grade, you can safely apply this massage oil throughout pregnancy—with better results than those achieved using traditional cocoa butter.

3 cups wheat germ oil

1 cup chopped fresh ginger root

1 cup chopped fresh turmeric root

In a double boiler, combine all of the ingredients. Bring to a simmer and heat for 30 minutes on medium-low heat.

Remove from heat and let cool to room temperature.

Strain through a cheesecloth or metal strainer to remove the ginger and turmeric pieces.

Massage into your skin twice a day.

Quick Tips

• Massaging stretch marks helps to increase blood flow to the area and improves healing.

• Apply tamanu oil (available at most health food and natural beauty stores) to stretch marks twice a day to increase the production of collagen and renew skin.

• It may not be your perfume of choice, but onion extract, with its anti-inflammatory and antibacterial properties, may help to regulate the formation of collagen when applied topically.

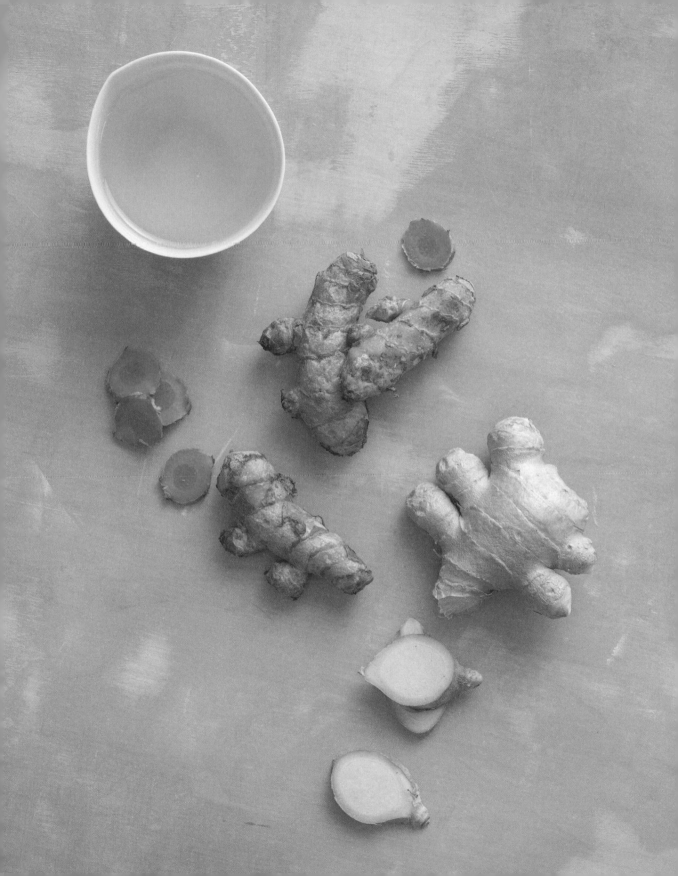

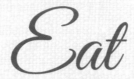

Eat

Food Cures
for Stretch Marks

When it comes to maintaining stretch-mark-free skin throughout your life, the keys are to increase the skin's elasticity before the fact and to boost collagen production and your body's healing processes after the fact. We all undergo growth spurts that leave our skin literally stretching to accommodate our changing bodies; but we don't need to endure the marks of an expanding body eternally.

With a diet rich in skin-healing vitamin E and zinc, as well as elasticity-boosting fats, fruit, and vegetables, you can prevent stretching skin from bearing the signs of a growth spurt and fade the marks of growths past.

As with pretty much anything, prevention is the best medicine. So, to newly pregnant women or girls just beginning puberty: if you anticipate the development of stretch marks and eat for more elastic skin from the inside out in advance, you can help to prevent them from ever setting up shop on your skin in the first place.

Sweet Green Smoothie

From Molly Sims, model and actress

Vegetarian, vegan, dairy-free, gluten-free, nut-free

What's the secret to Molly Sims's enviable beauty? It's partly this green smoothie, which she drinks both to speed her metabolism and support her skin's health. Loaded with vitamin- and nutrient-rich fruit and vegetables, this delicious fiber-packed smoothie will flush your body with healing nutrients and boost your body's hydration, making skin more supple, elastic, and resistant to stretch marks.

Don't be scared by all the vegetables in this smoothie. The carrots, apples, and banana in this blended drink make it surprisingly sweet.

Serves 1 to 2

½ **cup organic spinach**

1 **head organic romaine lettuce**

3 to 4 **stalks of celery**

2 **carrots**

2 **kale leaves, destemmed**

1 **apple**

½ **lemon, juiced**

Banana or another fruit of choice (optional)

Purée the spinach, lettuce, celery, carrots, kale, and apple with 2 cups of water in a blender until smooth.

Add the lemon juice and banana or other fruit, if desired, and continue to process until well combined.

Avocado, Watercress, + Cumin Salad

From Latham Thomas, MamaGlow.com and author of the book *Mama Glow*

Vegetarian, vegan, dairy-free, gluten-free, nut-free

Few people understand the nutrition needs of growing, stretching skin like maternity expert and holistic nutritionist Latham Thomas. This yummy salad is what the Mama Glow maven recommends for keeping stretch marks away. The key ingredient: avocado. Rich in monounsaturated fats, avocados are not only easily burned for energy; they help to keep the skin elastic and strong as it grows during pregnancy. Plus, they contain vitamins A, C, and E, and more than twice the potassium of a banana. It's guaranteed to make every *mama glow*!

Serves 4

2 **teaspoons cumin seeds**

1 **bunch watercress, chopped**

3 **large ripe avocadoes**

2 **tablespoons lemon juice**

2 **tablespoons extra-virgin olive oil**

Roast the cumin seeds in a dry skillet over medium heat. Remove and crush in a mortar and pestle.

Place the watercress on a large plate.

Pit, peel, and thinly slice the avocados and arrange on top of watercress.

Sprinkle with lemon and oil and garnish with roasted cumin.

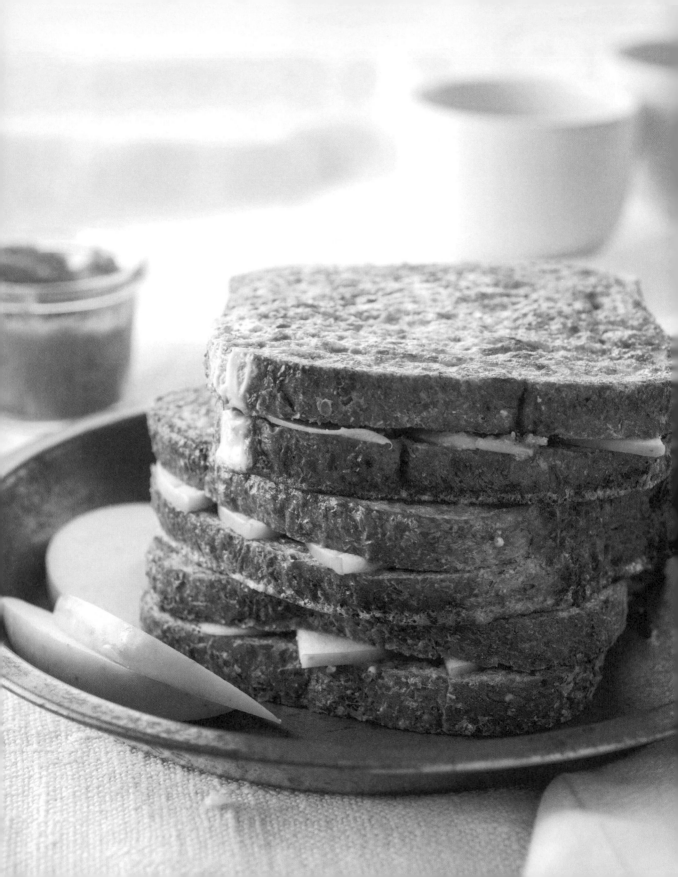

Grilled Nut Butter +
Apple Sandwich

Vegetarian

This dish is a stretch mark's worst enemy. The Brazil nuts this recipe calls for are high in zinc, a mineral essential for both collagen production and your body's wound-repairing processes. Sunflower seeds, pistachios, and almonds are high in vitamin E to support your body's ability to heal from the inside out. Slather this delicious nut butter spread on zinc-rich whole grain bread, add protein-packed eggs, and this irresistible sandwich will have you saying so-long to those stretch marks!

Serves 4

½ cup Brazil nuts

¼ cup raw pistachios

¼ cup raw almonds

1 cup raw sunflower seeds

3 tablespoons raw honey

Grape seed or almond oil,
     as needed

2 Granny Smith apples,
     thinly sliced

8 slices whole-wheat bread

2 eggs

In a blender, combine the nuts, seeds, and honey until a thick nut butter forms, approximately 2 to 4 minutes after the nuts are ground to a flour consistency. Slowly add the grape seed or almond oil, as needed, until your desired consistency develops. (You may need more of less depending on the speed, strength, and heat of your blender.)

Spread 1 to 2 tablespoons of the nut butter on each slice of bread.

Evenly divide the apple slices between 4 slices of bread, before topping with the other pieces of bread to create 4 sandwiches.

In a small bowl, whisk the eggs.

Lightly dip each sandwich in the egg wash, to coat on both sides, before placing on a greased frying pan on medium to high heat for about 30 seconds on each side, or until the bread crisps.

Quick Tips

• Vitamin E, found in nuts, seeds, and avocados, helps to protect and repair your skin's cell membranes.

• A little bit of self-tanner can help to conceal stretch marks until beauty recipes work their magic!

• Keep skin supple with a diet rich in fatty acids like those found in fish, olive oil, avocado, and hemp seeds.

• Massaging your skin helps to improve circulation, which, in turn, can prevent the appearance of stretch marks on growing skin.

Dry Skin + Rough Patches

When dry, drab, ashy skin is threatening to cramp your short-short-wearing, décolleté-displaying, back-baring sense of style, it's time to get serious. And I don't mean by investing in a new wardrobe that leaves little skin in sight or a lifetime supply of body lotion.

First, who has the money for a whole new wardrobe? Second, Every. Last. Drop. of body lotion that you put on your body gets absorbed into your skin. And have you read a lotion ingredient label lately? If you do, you're likely to prefer an all-natural solution for lackluster—or full-on drab—skin. With a few simple beauty recipes, you can take your skin from somber to sexy without the need for a chemical-full bottle of cream or a season spent hiding under layers of clothes.

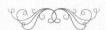

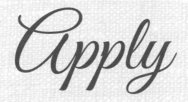

Apply

DIY Beauty Cures for
Dry Skin | Rough Patches

If you live in a dry climate, spend time in heated rooms, or travel frequently, dry skin may seem inevitable. But it's not. I do all three and can ensure you that a lifetime (or even a season) of dry skin that has you looking dull and feeling drab is easily escapable. Sure, there are some beauty products that brilliantly take skin from rough to radiant, but why go there when you can achieve the same results naturally, affordably, and easily—with just a quick trip to the grocery store.

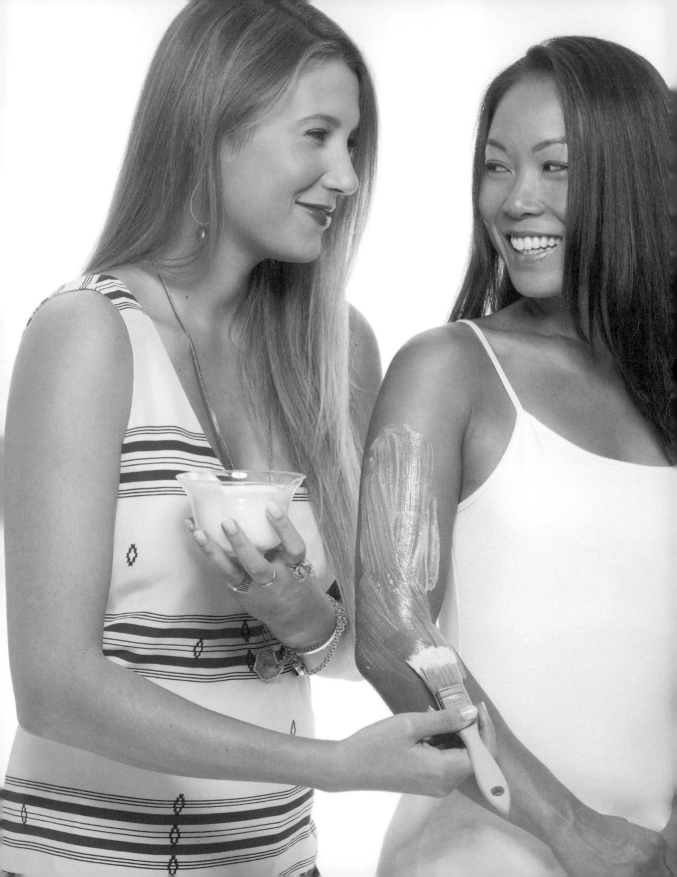

Baby Bottom Balm

All skin types

After fashion guru and creative director of *Elle*, Joe Zee, told me about the Beverly Hot Spring's milk, yogurt, and cucumber body-care treatment that he said made his skin "literally like a baby," I knew I had to DIY it. After grilling him for more info on the Los Angeles spa's treatment, I created this at-home recipe to give you (and me!) baby-like skin at home. With whole milk and yogurt, both of which have lactic acid to gently exfoliate and fat to moisturize, as well as cucumber, which is extremely hydrating, it's no wonder this body mask is Joe Zee's not-so-secret recipe for silky smooth skin.

½ cucumber, peeled and seeded
1 cup whole milk
2 cups plain full-fat yogurt
½ cup raw honey

In a food processor, purée the cucumber until smooth. Add the milk, yogurt, and honey and continue processing until well combined.

Using a pastry brush, apply a thin layer of the mask on any and all dry skin.

Let it sit for 10 to 15 minutes before rinsing with warm water.

Creamy Skin Treatment

All skin types

Brimming with beauty benefits because of their vitamin A, cholesterol, and fatty acids, egg yolks, when applied topically, heal dry skin and rough patches by gently exfoliating, healing, and hydrating—all at the same time. Mixed with lactic acid and protein-packed sour cream to gently exfoliate and restore skin's moisture, and avocado, with its especially hydrating fats, this recipe can take your skin from Sahara-like to silky smooth in no time. If skin is especially flaky, add honey for a more deeply penetrating effect.

1 avocado
3 egg yolks
2 tablespoons sour cream
2 tablespoons raw honey (optional)

In a small bowl, mash the inside of the avocado with a fork until smooth.

In a separate bowl, whisk the egg yolks.

Add the egg yolks, sour cream, and honey, if desired, to the avocado and mix until well combined.

Apply a thick layer to dry, dull skin and let it sit.

After 20 minutes, use a dry washcloth to scrub covered areas, exfoliating the softened skin.

Wash with warm water and pat dry.

Quick Tip

• Don't toss your avocado skins. Instead, rub the inside of an avocado peel on your body to exfoliate dry skin and hydrate with the bit of avocado left on the inside. Leave the residue on your skin for 5 minutes before rinsing in the shower and patting dry.

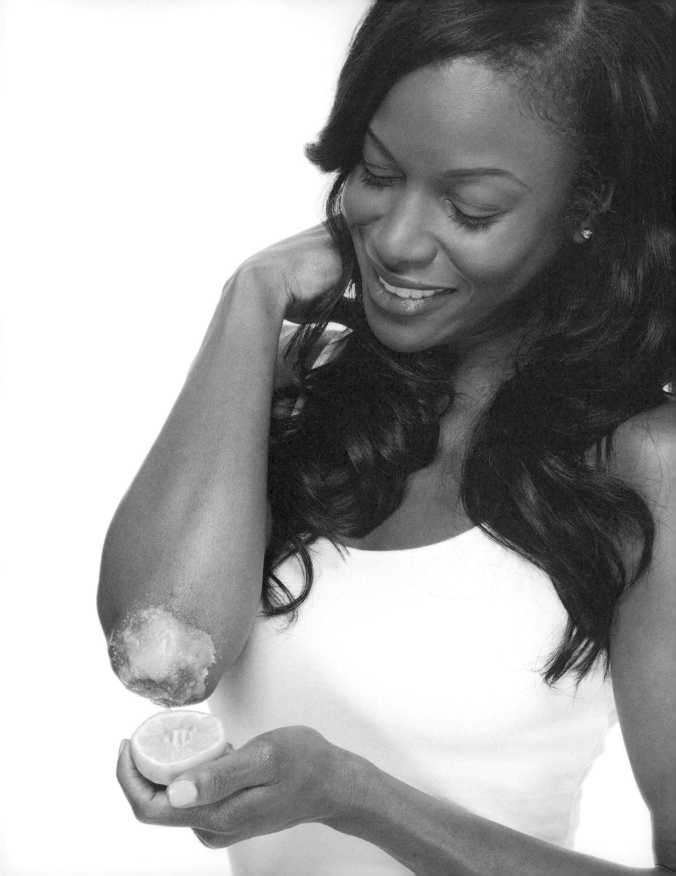

Lemonade
Lightening Scrub

Not for sensitive skin

Lemonade may already be a favorite of yours, but you're about to love it even more! With citric acid to break down dead, dull, dry skin and sugar to scrub it away, this easy at-home lemonade-like remedy is the ideal way to take skin from rough and rugged to soft and silky. It can help to fade age and sun spots, too, making it the perfect remedy for parched skin. Just remember, lemon juice can make you more sensitive to the sun and prone to burning, so use this at night and, as always, be sure to apply sunscreen before hitting the beach. While you're at it, whip up some lemonade too . . . you already have the ingredients!

1 lemon

¼ cup white sugar

1 tablespoon extra-virgin cold-pressed coconut oil

Cut the lemon in half. Squeeze about half of the juice from each half into a small bowl.

Rub the exposed side of the squeezed lemon halves on any dry, dull skin. (Don't be afraid to really dig your elbows, knees, or heels into the rind.)

Add sugar to the bowl with the lemon juice. Stir to combine, without letting the sugar melt.

On the area already primed with lemon juice, rub in the sugar mixture to scrub away dead, dry skin.

Rinse with warm water and pat dry before massaging skin with coconut oil.

"I do an olive oil and sugar scrub whenever I get chapped lips!"

—Emily Maynard, reality TV star, *The Bachelorette*

"I like to use grape seed oil as a moisturizer. It's inexpensive and keeps my skin looking glowy and feeling smooth."

—Amber Katz, BeautyBloggingJunkie.com

"Fill up the tub and pour in a ¹/₂ gallon of whole organic milk. Slather your body with raw honey before getting in the bath. Let the milk take the honey off. It definitely helps with dry skin. I got the idea from Cleopatra!"

—Kristina Anapau, actress

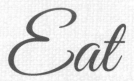

Eat

Food Cures for
Dry Skin + Rough Patches

Don't pick at your dry skin problem. Take a bite out of it—literally—with these recipes designed to work triple-duty. No matter the cause of your dehydrated skin, these recipes will help to speed up your body's process of both sloughing off dead, dry skin and producing new skin cells, while also encouraging your new skin cells to retain more moisture. With a diet rich in vitamin A, calcium, healthy fats, and water-dense fruit and vegetables, you can hydrate your skin from the inside out. The result: glowing skin you'll confidently flaunt, knowing it's soft, supple, and radiant.

Olive Oil Granola

Vegetarian, vegan, dairy-free, gluten-free

Loading up on healthy fats is one of the best ways to moisturize your skin from the inside out. A diverse array of nuts and seeds in this granola recipe each bring their own unique beauty benefit for soft, supple skin. With magnesium and vitamin K, cashews help to ensure adequate circulation and optimal absorption of calcium, which is essential for hydrated skin. Almonds, which are loaded with vitamin E, will help heal any skin damage, eczema, and psoriasis. Walnuts and flaxseeds, packed with über-moisturizing omega-3 fatty acids, ensure our skin stays hydrated. Pecans are the most antioxidant-dense nut, and sunflower seeds contain lignin phytoestrogens to prevent collagen breakdown and enhance the skin's lipid barrier. Altogether, this granola is like lotion in a bowl!

Serves 8

1 ½ cups gluten-free
  rolled oats

½ cup raw pistachios,
  shelled

⅓ cup raw pumpkin seeds

⅓ cup raw sunflower seeds

⅓ cup raw pecans

⅓ cup raw walnuts

⅓ cup raw almonds

⅓ cup raw cashews

½ cup unsweetened
  shredded coconut

1 teaspoon salt

2 tablespoons ground flaxseeds

⅓ cup extra-virgin olive oil

¼ cup agave

½ cup dried cranberries (fruit
  juice sweetened preferred)

Preheat the oven to 350°F.

In a large bowl, combine all of the dry ingredients except for the dried cranberries.

In a small bowl, combine the oil and agave.

Add the wet ingredients to the dry ingredients.

Spread the mixture evenly on a parchment-lined baking sheet. Bake for 40 minutes, stirring at 10 minute intervals to prevent burning.

Let cool to room temperature before stirring in dried cranberries. Store in an air-tight container.

Serve with soy milk, if desired—or just eat it straight out of the oven!

Quick Tip

• Your skin is one of the first places to show signs of dehydration. Drink 8 to 10 glasses of water and eat water-dense fruits and vegetables to keep your skin soft and supple.

Kale Chips + Spicy Cucumber Dip

Vegetarian, gluten-free, nut-free

Kale just may be the queen of greens. Just one cup contains 180 percent of the daily requirement of vitamin A, which your body needs to turn over dry skin; 200 percent of vitamin C, which protects skin from environmental damage and dryness; and 1,020 percent of vitamin K, which helps to ensure optimal circulation—all of which work to ensure your body is healthy, hydrated, and protected from the inside out. Served with an avocado, cucumber, and yogurt-based dip for their moisturizing fats, firming silica, and hydrating calcium, respectively, and these kale chips are both tasty and a lot more beautifying than your usual chips and dip!

Serves 2 to 4

KALE CHIPS

1 bunch lacinato kale

3 tablespoons extra-virgin
   olive oil

1 teaspoon coarse salt
   (optional)

SPICY CUCUMBER DIP

1 avocado

½ English cucumber, with skin

⅓ cup Greek yogurt

1 tablespoon lime juice

½ teaspoon kosher salt

2 tablespoons fresh mint, diced

1 jalapeño pepper, chopped

For the Kale Chips

Preheat the oven to 350°F.

Wash and dry kale leaves before tossing with oil to evenly coat.

Place kale in an even layer on a baking sheet. Sprinkle with salt, if desired.

Bake for 15 minutes, or until crispy.

Transfer to a paper towel to cool and absorb excess oil.

For the Spicy Cucumber Dip

In a food processor, combine all of the ingredients except jalapeño until smooth.

Slowly add jalapeño until desired heat is achieved. If your dip gets too spicy, add more lime to cut the heat.

Serve immediately.

Quick Tip

• Silica, found in cucumber peel, helps hydrate your skin and maintain elasticity—so keep the peel on your cucumbers from now on!

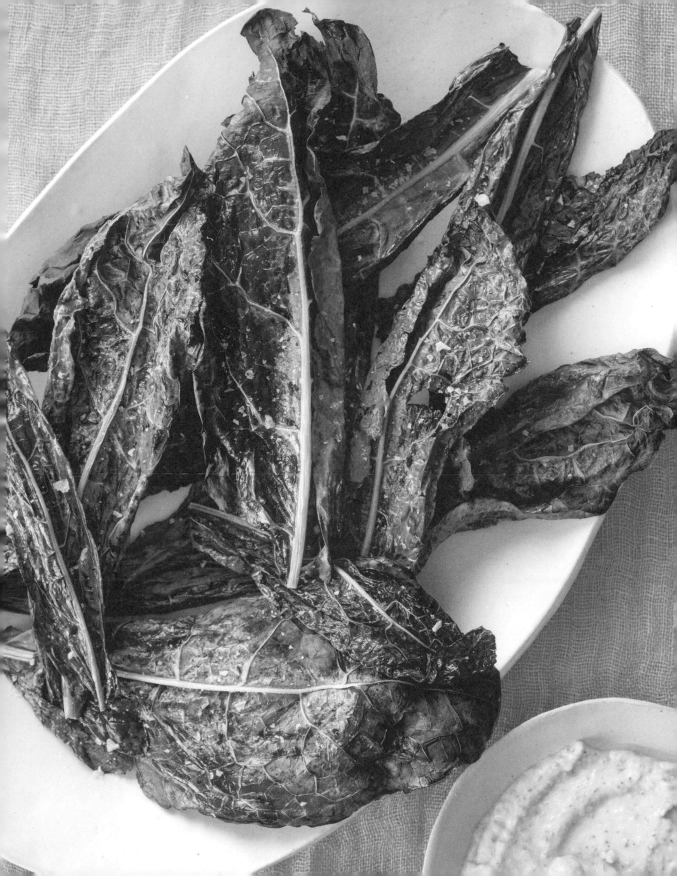

Honey Roasted
Delicata Squash Salad

From Manuel Trevino, *Top Chef* contestant

Vegetarian, gluten-free

Delicata squash, with its telltale dark green stripes, may have less skin-saving beta-carotene and exfoliating vitamin A than other squash varieties, but its potassium content, which helps keep skin hydrated, more than makes up for it. Combined with the healthy fats of the hazelnuts and olive oil, as well as the calcium and protein of the burrata, this salad is sure to help keep your skin hydrated from the inside out.

Serves 2 to 4

1 delicata squash

4 tablespoons honey

Salt and pepper, to taste

2 ounces arugula

4 tablespoons pomegranate seeds

4 tablespoons vincotto

4 tablespoons extra-virgin olive oil

4 tablespoons hazelnuts, toasted

8 ounces burrata

Preheat the oven to 375°F.

Peel and cut the squash in half. Scoop out the seeds and cut the squash into ¼-inch half moons.

Toss the squash with the honey, salt, and pepper and roast until tender, about 6 to 8 minutes.

Combine the arugula, squash, and pomegranate seeds. Dress with the vincotto and oil. Top with the toasted hazelnuts and a large piece of burrata.

Quick Tip
• Calcium deficiencies can lead to dry skin so make sure you're eating enough calcium-rich dairy products and/or dark green leafy vegetables.

Donna Karan's Daily Green Juice

From Donna Karan, fashion designer and founder of Urban Zen

Vegetarian, vegan, dairy-free, gluten-free, nut-free

Few people radiate beauty from the inside out quite like Donna Karan. Her incredible talent, drive, and enormous heart (as evidenced by her founding of the Urban Zen foundation) are barely matched by her radiant complexion. Her glow is due in part to her daily green juice recipe. Donna says, "I drink this green juice every day. It's one of the ways that I nurture and take care of myself. To me, that's beautiful." I'm thrilled she shared it with me—and now you! Loaded with hydrating and skin-protecting fruit and vegetables, a daily dose of this green juice will keep your skin protected from free radicals and hydrated from the inside out.

For best results, all ingredients should be organic and/or locally grown and juice should be consumed within a couple of days to reap the benefits of the live enzymes.

Serves 8

6 to 8 large romaine leaves

4 to 6 leaves lacinato kale

2 Granny Smith apples

4 Fuji apples

1 bulb of fennel

½ head celery

1 cucumber

1 yellow pepper

12 ounces baby spinach

1 piece of ginger, 1-inch thick

1 lemon

In a large bowl, soak the romaine and kale leaves in cold water. Gently stir the leaves to help remove the sand and then lift the leaves out of the water and place in a clean bowl.

Wash the rest of the fruit and vegetables in cold water.

Cut all of the fruit and vegetables into small pieces that will easily fit into the mouth of your juicer.

Using a juicer, proceed to juice all of the ingredients, alternating between the leafy vegetables and the fruit. Store in the refrigerator for up to 2 days.

Quick Tip

• Not into fish? Get your omega-3 fatty acids from chia seeds! Sprinkle on salads or in smoothies for their hydrating benefits.

Uneven Skin Tone + Texture (+ Self-Tanner Mishaps!)

At some point in your life you will notice uneven skin tone. It's not an "if," it's a "when." It even happens to the best of us—and by "best of us," I mean those of us who apply SPF religiously and take care of our bodies inside and out. If your skin is uneven in tone or texture due to natural or environmental causes, like hormonal changes or too much time spent in the sun, there's a recipe here for you. And because the same factors that lead to uneven skin tone—dry, not-nearly-as-exfoliated-as-necessary skin—also cause your self-tanner to apply and fade unevenly, each recipe here also works to fix self-tanner mishaps.

So, next time you're gearing up for bikini season or prepping for some other scantily clad activity (no judgments!), start here to ensure you're smooth and even from shoulder to soles.

Please note, for uneven skin on your face, turn back to Chapter 1, as the APPLY recipes here are too abrasive for your delicate face, neck, and décolleté.

Apply

DIY Beauty Cures
for Uneven Skin Tone + Texture
(+ Self-Tanner Mishaps!)

Whether your uneven skin tone is caused by permanent-until-now hyperpigmentation or a botched self-tanner job, the solution is the same: to break down the dead, darkened skin cells and then exfoliate them away. Relying on both chemical and manual exfoliants to break down the stickiness of your skin cells and then scrub them away, respectively, these beauty recipes work wonders.

While you'll see improvement with each of these immediately, results are cumulative, so don't give up if your skin isn't instantly flawless. And remember: the sooner you treat your skin, the more effective these remedies are, so stop waiting and get cooking.

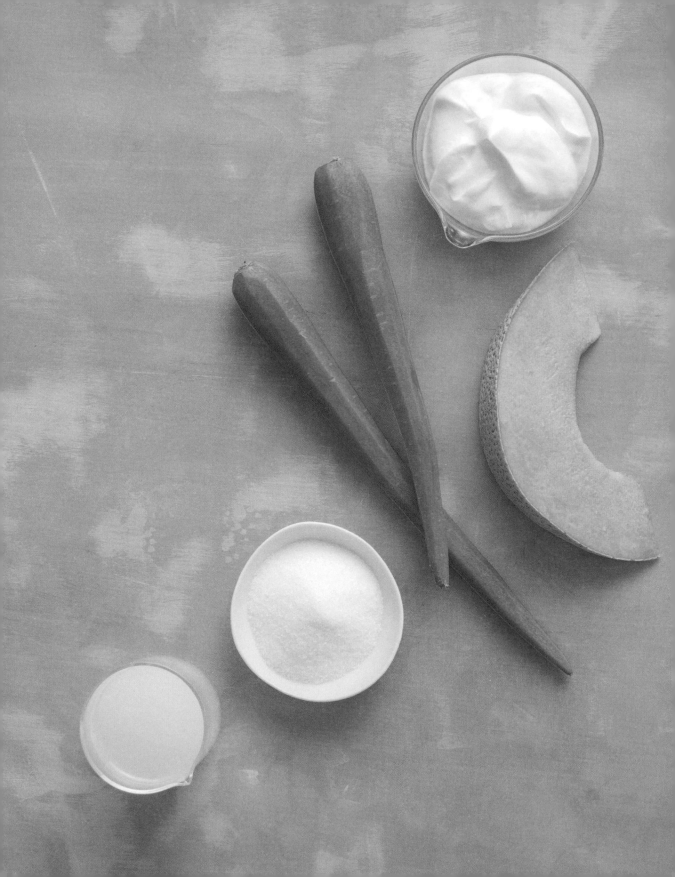

Cantaloupe + Carrot
Illuminating Mask

All skin types

What if you could get the exfoliating benefits of retinols, a chemical peel, and an exfoliating scrub all in one? With this mask, you (sort of) can. Carrots and cantaloupe are both rich in vitamin A, the key ingredient in prescription retinols. Yogurt and lemon juice have chemical-peel regulars lactic and citric acid, respectively; and sugar, as you probably know by now, is a great exfoliator. With all these ingredients, this mask-meets-scrub is just what your uneven skin tone is hungry for. And, considering it's all food-based, you can snack on it too, if you'd like.

¼ **cup carrots**

¼ **cup cantaloupe**

½ **cup plain yogurt**

1 **tablespoon lemon juice**

¼ **cup white sugar**

Steam the carrots until fork tender. Drain and refrigerate until cool, about 2 hours.

Once chilled, in a food processor, combine the carrots, cantaloupe, yogurt, and lemon juice. Purée until smooth.

Transfer to a mixing bowl before stirring in the sugar.

Massage over your hyperpigmented areas for at least 5 minutes.

Let the mixture sit on your skin to penetrate for an additional 10 to 15 minutes before rinsing with warm water.

Quick Tip

• Picking at blemishes can lead to long-term discoloration. Step away from the mirror and don't even think about squeezing that pimple!

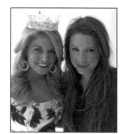

When self-tanner application goes awry, what does a beauty queen do? "I mix sugar and salt together and a little olive oil—and scrub all over."

—Mallory Hagan, Miss America 2013

Margarita Brightening Scrub

Not for acne-prone or irritated skin

When your skin is unevenly colored or textured and not homogenizing on its own (or at least not quickly enough for you), why not help it along? With a combination of citric acid from the lime juice to help break down dead skin cells and salt to help scrub it all away, this recipe will help to gently and effectively exfoliate away hyperpigmented skin that's near the surface. Even better, the vitamin C in the lime juice and vitamin E in the olive oil work together to help put your body's natural healing—and evening—processes into overdrive, to gradually reduce the appearance of deeper dark spots over time. And the tequila? It's an antiseptic, helping to ensure your skin is clean, clear, and ready for scrubbing!

¼ **cup white tequila**

3 **tablespoons lime juice**

¼ **cup extra-virgin olive oil**

¼ **cup apple cider vinegar**

½ **cup sea salt**

Combine the tequila, lime juice, oil, and vinegar, whisking until as well combined as possible. Stir in the salt.

After a warm bath or shower, on damp, softened skin, apply the mixture in gentle circular motions. On the thicker skin on your body (like elbows and heels), use a washcloth for a more aggressive scrub, if desired.

Briefly rinse with warm water, leaving residual oil on your skin to moisturize.

Lightening Overnight Toner

All skin types

Vitamin C not only protects your skin from the environmental causes of uneven skin tone and texture, it also helps to reverse past damage by breaking down your skin's melanin (the substance responsible for your skin's color), thereby reducing hyperpigmentation. With the highest concentration of vitamin C in any fruit, guava makes an ideal treatment for dark spots. Paired with lemon juice, which is both a great source of vitamin C and packed with citric acid to help break down darkened skin cells, this toner (when used regularly), will even out skin tone and texture, naturally.

1 **guava, peeled**

4 **tablespoons lemon juice**

In a blender, purée the guava and lemon juice until smooth.

Use a cotton swab to apply a thin layer to cleansed, hyperpigmented areas at bedtime.

Quick Tip

• The #1 way to prevent hyperpigmentation is with SPF! Apply it daily to help prevent skin discoloration from happening in the first place.

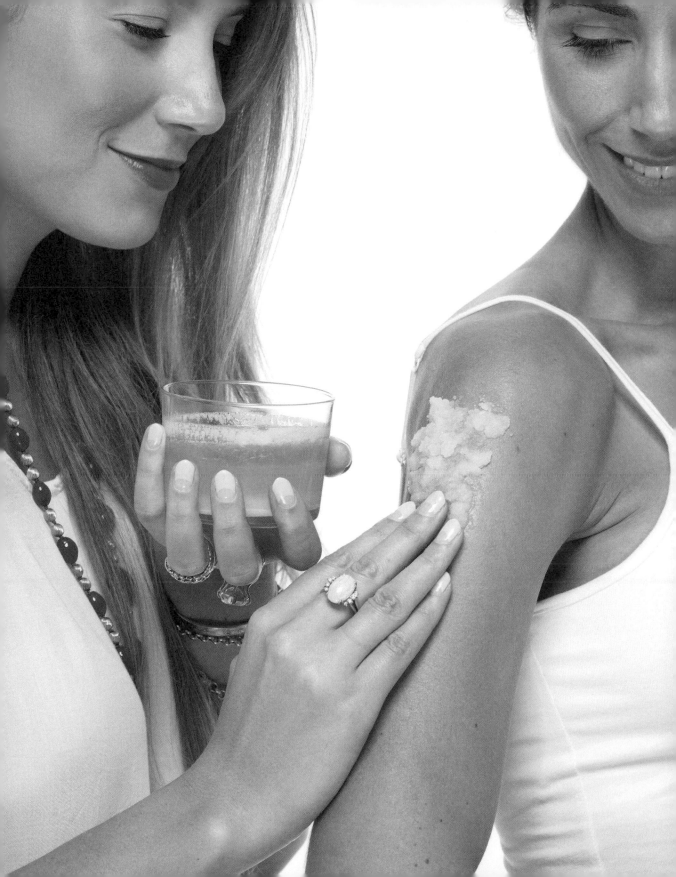

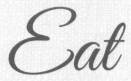

Eat

Food Cures for Uneven Skin Tone + Texture (+ Self-Tanner Mishaps!)

Damaged skin, whether discolored or unevenly textured, is just one bite away from a solution. Okay, maybe a lot of bites away, but you get the idea! By eating a diet densely packed with lycopene, vitamin E, omega-3 fatty acids, protein, vitamin A, selenium, copper, and manganese, you feed your body with all it needs to heal itself and its currently less-than-flawless skin from the inside out. The result: skin that's healed from past damage and protected from further hyperpigmentation and uneven texture.

Charred Red Pepper Dip

Vegetarian, vegan, dairy-free, gluten-free

Studies have shown that lycopene, found in red peppers, helps smooth unevenly textured skin and protects our bodies from the harmful effects of UV sun damage, all from the inside out. Also containing vitamin-E rich sesame seeds and omega-3 fatty acid-packed walnuts, this dip will help to ensure a healthy, even complexion from head to toe.

Serves 4

2 red bell peppers
½ cup walnuts
2 tablespoons tahini
½ teaspoon honey
2 teaspoons red wine vinegar
½ teaspoon cumin
¼ teaspoon cayenne
½ teaspoon salt
½ teaspoon sweet red or
  white wine (optional)
Black pepper, to taste

Broil the whole peppers on high, turning occasionally, until evenly charred, about 10 minutes.

Toast the walnuts in a dry skillet until slightly browned and fragrant.

When the peppers are done, let them sit until cooled enough to remove and discard the seeds and skins.

In a food processor, combine the peppers, walnuts, tahini, honey, vinegar, cumin, cayenne, salt, and wine, if desired. Purée until smooth. Season with fresh ground black pepper, to taste.

Serve with cucumber slices or whole grain chips or spread on sandwiches instead of mayonnaise.

Quick Tip

• Encouraging cell turnover may be the best way to fade dark spots, but it also makes your skin more susceptible to further sun damage, so be sure to use SPF daily (I can't encourage this enough!).

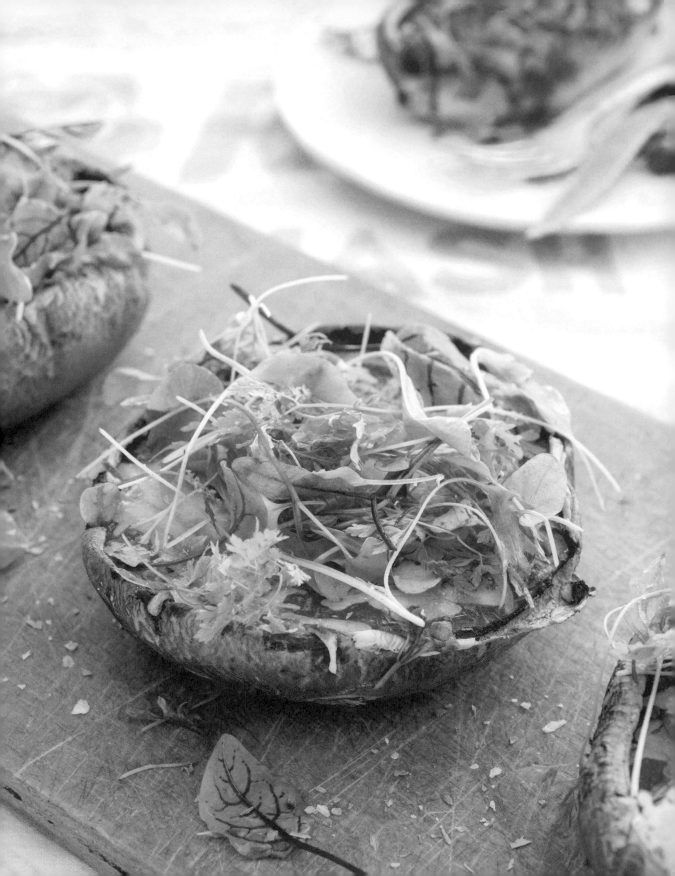

Portobello Mushroom "Pizza" + Mesclun Greens

From Amanda K. Walley, personal chef and owner of Tortured Orchard Seasoning Sauces

Vegetarian, gluten-free, nut-free

For most of us, uneven skin tone, if not directly caused by sun damage, is most definitely exacerbated by it. Adding more lycopene-rich foods, like tomatoes, to your diet, can help protect your skin from the sun's rays. A study out of the United Kingdom actually found that subjects eating a high-lycopene diet for three months increased their sun protection by 33 percent!

There's a correlation between lycopene and skin texture, too, meaning that the tomato sauce in this "pizza" will not only prevent the sun from discoloring your skin but will simultaneously help to smooth your unevenly textured skin. Combined with selenium-packed mushrooms, which protect skin quality, support optimal elasticity, and further reduce sun damage, it's safe to consider this a guilt-free pizza!

Serves 1

- 1 portobello mushroom
- 3 to 4 tablespoons marinara sauce
- 2 tablespoons part-skim mozzarella cheese
- 1 tablespoon pecorino romano cheese
- 1 tablespoon parmesan cheese
- Pinch of dried oregano
- Pinch of garlic powder
- Pinch of cracked black pepper
- ¾ cup mesclun greens
- 1 tablespoon balsamic vinegar
- 1 teaspoon extra-virgin olive oil

Preheat the oven to 450°F.

Wipe the mushroom free of dirt with a damp towel. Remove and discard the stem and gills (the brown matter under the cap). Saving the cap, turn it over so the mushroom resembles a bowl.

Fill the mushroom with the sauce and cheeses, sprinkling the top of the cheeses with the oregano, garlic powder, and pepper. Once assembled, your mushroom should resemble a little individual pizza.

Place the "pizza" on a tinfoil-lined cookie sheet and bake for 20 minutes, or until the cheese is melted and slightly browned.

In a small mixing bowl, combine salad greens with vinegar and oil. Once the mushroom is out of the oven, let it cool for 1 to 2 minutes before plating and topping with mixed greens.

Blueberry Crustless Quiche

Vegetarian, gluten-free, nut-free

Next time you're craving a blueberry muffin, try this instead! Protein-packed and loaded with skin-saving vitamin A, eggs (especially the yolks!) are one of the best beauty-boosting foods for your skin, helping it to look radiant and smooth. Help heal your skin from the inside out with spinach, which is full of iron, vitamin A, and vitamin E, and encourage smoother, firmer, more supple skin with blueberries, which boost collagen production. With this delectable quiche, breakfast just got more beautiful, in more ways than one. P.S. You won't even taste the spinach!

Serves 6

4 cups spinach, packed

12 eggs

6 cups fresh blueberries, divided

1 ½ cups maple syrup

1 ½ cups cottage cheese

Preheat the oven to 350°F.

Purée the spinach in a food processor.

Scramble the eggs before mixing with the spinach.

In a non-stick muffin pan, place ¼ cup of the blueberries in the bottom of each of 12 muffin cups. Top each with the egg and spinach mixture until ¾ full. Bake for 25 to 30 minutes or until set.

In a small sauce pan, sauté the remaining blueberries with the maple syrup over low heat until the berries burst, about 5 to 7 minutes. Remove from heat and stir in cottage cheese. Serve over quiche.

Quick Tip
• SPF is like body armor against sun spots. If you can see your hand in front of your face, you need sunscreen. Yes, even at dusk. Yes, even in the winter.

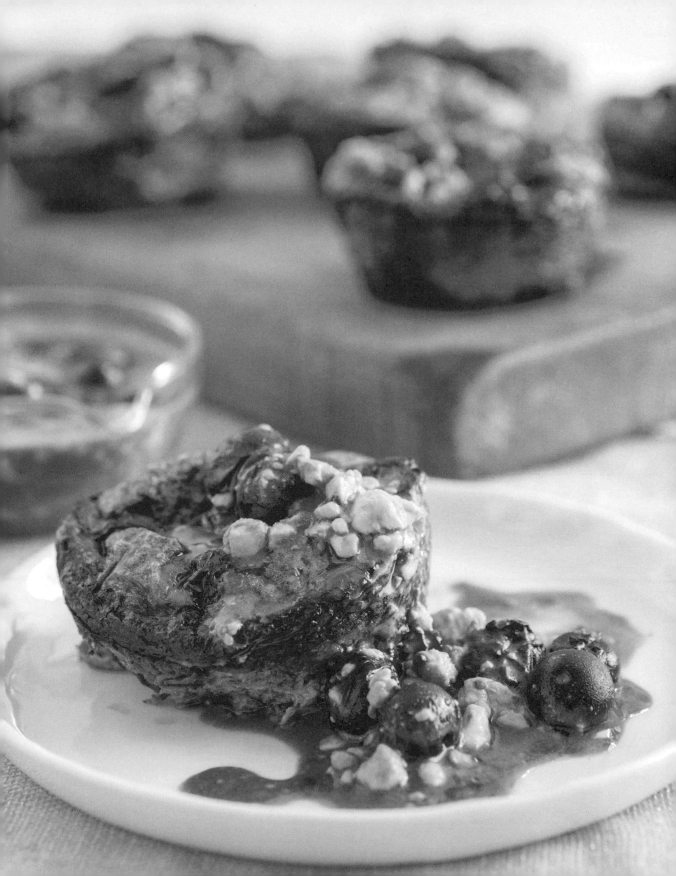

Grilled Pineapple with Cashew Butter + Vanilla Frozen Yogurt

From Alexandra Ray, pastry chef at North End Grill, New York City

Vegetarian, gluten-free

Pineapple, packed with vitamin C and manganese, helps to reduce inflammation, improve skin texture, and keep skin even while simultaneously ensuring that your body is able to metabolize the vitamins designed to improve skin tone. Meanwhile, cashews are rich in copper, a trace mineral that's essential for wound-healing (yes, your uneven skin tone is, technically speaking, a "wound"). Together these beautifying ingredients make a decadent dessert—so move over Ben & Jerry's!

Serves 8

1 pineapple

1 ½ tablespoons chopped ginger

¾ cup dark brown sugar

½ cup mint syrup

24 mint leaves, cut in long, thin strips

½ teaspoon ground black pepper

½ teaspoon ground toasted coriander

1 teaspoon kosher salt, divided

½ vanilla bean

2 cups cashews

½ teaspoon kosher salt

3 tablespoons + 2 teaspoons grape seed oil

4 cups vanilla frozen yogurt

Cut the skin off the pineapple by first removing both ends and then going down the sides with a sharp knife to cut off the spiny skin. Slice the pineapple into ½-inch pieces.

In a mixing bowl, combine ginger, brown sugar, mint syrup, mint leaves, black pepper, coriander, ½ teaspoon salt, and vanilla bean. Add ⅓ cup and 2 tablespoons of water.

Marinate the pineapple slices in the mixture overnight.

Toast the cashews in a dry skillet until golden brown.

Place the cashews and the remaining salt in a food processor. Slowly add the grape seed oil and process until the butter is smooth. Set aside.

Strain the pineapple slices, reserving the marinade to serve as a sauce.

Light the grill.

Rinse the marinade off the pineapple slices and grill, creating char marks on both sides.

Heat the marinade over low heat.

Cut pineapple slices, as desired, and serve with a smear of the cashew butter. Top with the vanilla frozen yogurt and the marinade.

Ingrown Hairs + Razor Burn

Assuming you're one of the 99 percent of women (well, women reading this book anyway) who remove body hair from at least some part of your body on a regular basis, you've likely had an ingrown hair or razor burn or both . . . sometimes simultaneously . . . in a "Are the hair removal gods really this evil?" kind of way.

You know what I'm talking about: those red or dark, sometimes painful, always unsightly pimple-like gnarlies that always show up at the worst possible moment. As in, just after you've done the pre-sex emergency bikini shave, which you immediately regret because a little stubble is infinitely better than a vagina that, best-case scenario, looks ravaged by a rash or, worst-case, appears to be where the measles, mumps, and rubella plague went to die. Not that I actually know what any of those look like, but you get the picture!

When it comes to the hair on our bodies we're looking to remove, there are two common beauty problems that (all too often) appear: ingrown hairs and razor burn— a serious misnomer, by the way, because similar irritation can appear post-wax, too.

Razor burn is the immediate reaction to a less-than-lubricated shave or too-harsh-wax. While ingrown hairs, much as the name implies, are when a previously plucked, shaved, or waxed hair is attempting to grow back in but instead gets trapped within a clogged pore, under the surface of your skin. Sexy, huh?

Sure, an easy way to prevent both razor burn and ingrown hairs would be to stop removing the hair in the first place. But assuming you're not looking to tap into your inner unkempt flower child (as endearing as a throwback to the '70s may seem), keep reading for some all-natural solutions that will ensure your hoo-ha, under-arms, and well, any other area you're currently removing hair from are as smooth as a baby's hairless bottom.

Apply

DIY Beauty Cures for Ingrown Hairs + Razor Burn

If you are a chronic sufferer of ingrown hairs or razor burn:

A: Change your hair removal method. Waxing and shaving affect each of us differently. For some women, waxing is more irritating, while for others shaving is more problematic.

B: Keep reading, because with my APPLY and EAT secrets, you'll have effective fixes for both issues.

The solution here is two-fold. First, to prevent immediately occurring irritation post-shave or wax (those small bumps that appear right after hair removal) and second, to ensure removed hairs can grow in unobstructed (i.e., in-grown free).

Pre-Shave Oil

All skin types

If your current shaving cream or gel isn't keeping you smooth and razor-burn free, pre-shave oil could be the solution for you. While some men have already jumped on this bandwagon to prevent razor-burn and ingrown hairs on their faces, when it comes to shaving our legs, underarms, bikini lines, or anywhere else, women seem (uncharacteristically, of course) to be a step behind.

This pre-shave oil recipe contains safflower oil, rich in anti-inflammatory linoleic acid, and coconut oil, for its antimicrobial lauric acid. This duo of oils softens the skin (so it's more pliable) and hair (so it's less likely to snag) and helps keep redness, inflammation, and infection at bay, for a closer, smoother, and irritation-and-ingrown-hair-free shave.

1 tablespoon extra-virgin cold-pressed coconut oil, liquefied

1 tablespoon safflower oil

Combine the oils in a small bowl.

Apply a warm washcloth to the area to be shaved for 5 minutes. Massage the oil mixture into the area. Let it sit for 10 minutes. Cover with another warmed towel for an additional 5 minutes. Shave immediately.

Adjust measurements, as needed, depending on the size of the area to be shaved.

Quick Tips

• Add 2 to 3 drops of tea tree oil to 1 tablespoon of olive oil and massage into skin that is irritated by razor burn to kill bacteria and moisturize.

• As they help for a cyst-like pimple, warm compresses will open the pore, allowing a trapped hair to come to the surface.

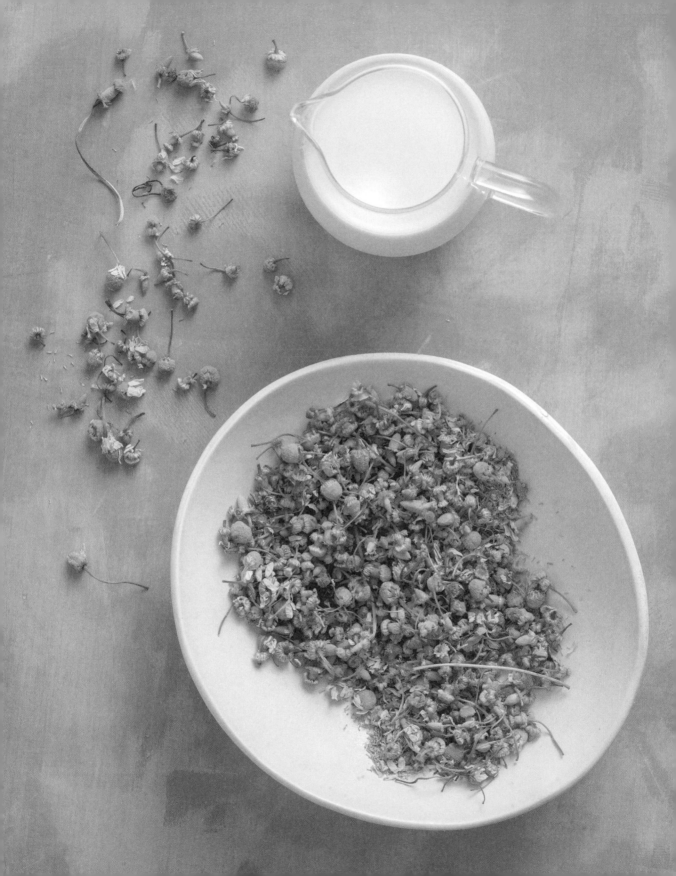

Skin Soothing
After Shave

All skin types

Men use aftershave on their faces, so why aren't you using it on your body, too? Maybe because you don't want to smell like a man? Well, now you don't have to. With a homemade after-shave toner made with gently exfoliating milk and calming chamomile tea, you can prevent both inflammation and ingrown hairs, naturally and without smelling masculine. Plus, unlike most store-bought aftershaves loaded with alcohols, which dry out, irritate, and inflame the skin, this one is alcohol-free!

1 cup whole milk

4 bags chamomile tea

Warm the milk over low heat, stirring constantly. When hot, but not boiling, add the chamomile tea bags, cover, and let simmer for 15 minutes.

Remove from heat.

Discard the tea bags before pouring the chamomile milk into an ice cube tray and freezing.

After shaving, rub one cube over the shaved area to reduce redness and irritation, close pores, and prevent ingrown hairs.

Quick Tips

• If you currently have an ingrown hair, you can use the warm tea bags as a compress to open the pore, reduce inflammation, and encourage exfoliation, before discarding.

• A sharp razor will reduce the likelihood of irritation, so change your razor blade often.

Daily Exfoliating Scrub

Not for sensitive skin

One of the best ways to prevent ingrown hairs from setting up shop on your usually soft, smooth skin is to exfoliate regularly. When used daily (or at least prior to shaving or waxing), this scrub will ensure no hairs get trapped under a layer of dead skin cells, wreaking havoc in their attempt to reach the surface. With the lactic acid in the milk to calm your skin and gently chemically exfoliate, two types of sugars to manually exfoliate, and honey to kill bacteria and moisturize, your skin will be silky smooth in no time.

½ cup whole milk

¼ cup raw honey

½ cup white sugar

¼ cup sugar in the raw

Combine all of the ingredients in a small bowl.
On clean, damp, warm skin (ideally during or after a shower), apply the mixture in gentle circular motions to exfoliate skin.
Rinse with warm water and pat dry.

Quick Tips

• A severe ingrown hair sometimes requires professional intervention. See a dermatologist if an ingrown hair is cyst-like for more than a couple of days.

• Exfoliate 24 hours before waxing to make the shorter hairs easier to grip.

"I'm one of those 'blessed' with having to shave every day, and the constant shaving friction and detergents in body washes can make my legs feel itchy and dry. I've found the best solution is to use organic coconut oil in place of shaving gel on my legs. Coconut oil is replete with vitamin E and a deep concentration of over 90 percent healthy fat, so it gives your legs a resuscitative, moisturizing treatment while you're shaving. Depending on your skin type and the season, you may not even need lotion after you hop out of the shower!"

—Grace Gold, beauty journalist

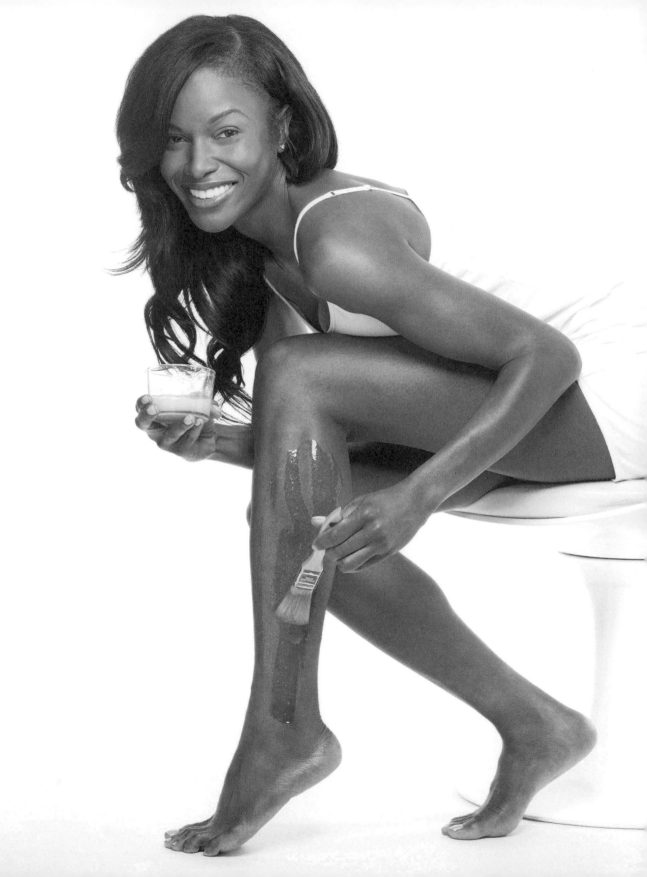

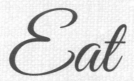

Eat

Food Cures for
Ingrown Hairs + Razor Burn

More often than not, an ingrown hair is the result of skin that's either dry, not exfoliated enough or, more often than not, both, leading to dead skin cells that clog the pore and trap the hair below the surface. (Gross, I know, but thankfully they're about to be a thing of the past.) To prevent ingrown hairs from setting up shop on your skin in the first place, you need to do two things: 1) Ensure that your skin is hydrated so dry skin doesn't clog pores. 2) Make sure your skin is optimally exfoliating itself so those dead skin cells don't block hairs from growing in freely.

These same solutions will also help to keep skin soft and smooth for a less irritating shave and fewer post-shave or -wax bumps and bruises, too. In case that's still not enough, these recipes will also help to keep inflammation at bay, so in the off chance you still experience some post-hair removal irritation from a wax gone awry or an ingrown hair from a shave done in haste, you can rest assured that redness and inflammation will be minimal at most (and nonexistent at best).

Tropical Popeye

From Matthew Kenney, chef

Vegetarian, vegan, dairy-free, gluten-free, nut-free

Keep skin soft, supple, and irritation-free with a daily dose of this smoothie recipe from famed raw food chef Matthew Kenney. With anti-inflammatory ginger and aloe, hydrating coconut butter and coconut water; and vitamin-packed spinach and pineapple, this sweet, green smoothie will both prevent irritation from shaving or waxing and reduce the discomfort and unsightliness of existing razor burn or ingrown hairs.

Serves 1 to 2

1 ¾ cups pineapple, cubed

1 ½ cups spinach

2 thin slices of ginger

2 tablespoons coconut butter

2 tablespoons 100% pure aloe vera gel or juice

½ tablespoon agave

½ cup coconut water

Pinch of sea salt

Place all the ingredients in a high-powered blender and purée until smooth. Serve immediately.

Turmeric Dip

Vegetarian, vegan, dairy-free, gluten-free, nut-free

If you're not only prone to ingrown hairs, but also unlucky enough for them to be unsightly, extremely red, raised, and painful, this dip is for you. With turmeric, this dip will reduce inflammation while simultaneously helping to keep bacteria away. With such powerful anti-inflammatory benefits, this dip can also help to relieve bruising from waxing, or anything else—like when you try to balance on one leg while shaving in the shower and it doesn't go as well as planned (or am I the only one without any yoga-shower skills to speak of?)!

Serves 6 to 8

1 cup raw cashews, soaked

1 tablespoon extra-virgin olive oil

2 cloves garlic

¼ cup coconut milk

1 tablespoon turmeric

1 teaspoon ginger

1 tablespoon agave

Carrot sticks, to serve

Cucumber slices, to serve

Cover the cashews in water and soak for at least 3 hours.

Drain the cashews and transfer to a food processor. Add the olive oil, garlic, coconut milk, turmeric, ginger, and agave and process until smooth.

Serve with carrot sticks and cucumber slices.

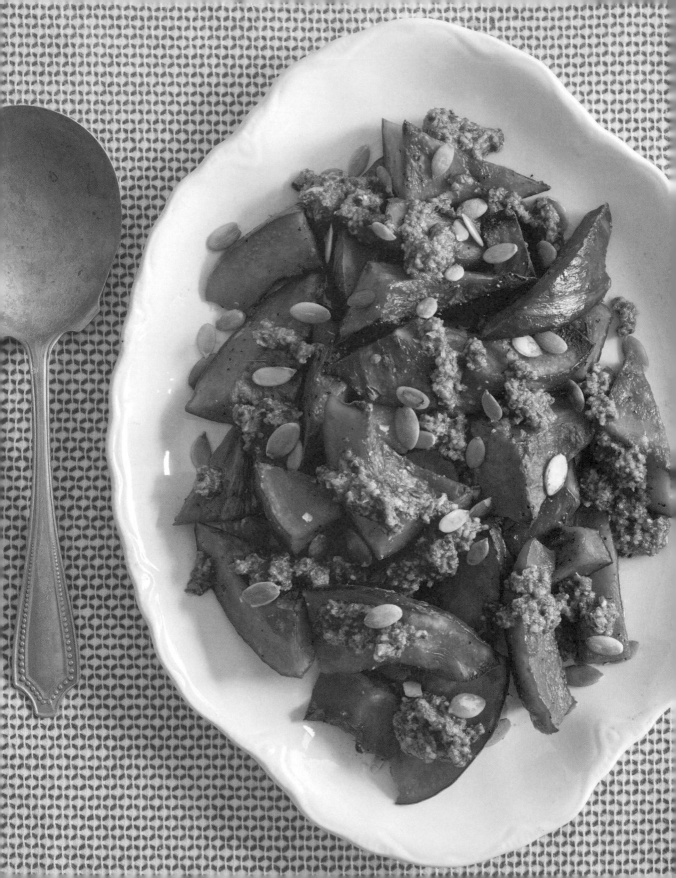

Kabocha Squash with Walnut Pesto

Vegetarian, gluten-free

Kabocha squash may be less well known than its "squash sisters," but with 70 percent of your recommended daily amount of vitamin A in a single serving, this low-carb Japanese squash packs quite a punch against ingrown hairs by preventing clogged pores from the inside out. It's served with pesto, which has antibacterial and hydrating properties from its basil and nuts, respectively. Add magnesium-rich pumpkin seeds, which help to improve circulation and this hearty antioxidant and anti-inflammatory squash is like kryptonite for congested skin.

Serves 2 to 4

ROASTED KABOCHA SQUASH

- 1 medium kabocha squash
- 1 tablespoon extra-virgin cold-pressed coconut oil, melted
- ¼ teaspoon sea salt
- ¼ teaspoon black pepper

WALNUT PESTO

- 3 tablespoons raw pumpkin seeds
- ⅓ cup + 2 tablespoons extra-virgin olive oil, divided
- ½ teaspoon sea salt, divided
- 2 tablespoons raw pine nuts
- 1 garlic clove, sliced
- 1 cup fresh basil, tightly packed
- 2 tablespoons raw walnuts
- ¼ teaspoon lemon juice
- ½ cup freshly grated Parmesan cheese

For the Roasted Kabocha Squash

Preheat the oven to 400°F.

Cut off the top and bottom of the kabocha squash and discard before cutting it in half and scooping out and discarding the seeds and fibrous center. Cut into 1 to 2-inch wedges.

Toss the squash with the coconut oil and sprinkle with the salt and pepper.

Place the squash in a single layer on a baking sheet and bake for 30 minutes, flipping half way through.

For the Walnut Pesto

Place the pumpkin seeds and 1 tablespoon of the olive oil in a skillet over medium heat and cook, stirring constantly, until lightly toasted. Sprinkle with ¼ teaspoon sea salt and set aside.

In the same skillet, put 1 tablespoon olive oil, pine nuts, and garlic and cook, stirring constantly, until the pine nuts are lightly toasted. Transfer to a food processor.

Add remaining olive oil, basil, walnuts, lemon juice, cheese, and salt and process until smooth.

Top cooked kabocha with fresh pesto and toasted pumpkin seeds before serving.

Quick Tip

- Prevent clogged pores from leading to ingrown hairs by eating more foods high in vitamin A (like sweet potatoes, squash, and dark green leafy vegetables), which support your body's natural exfoliation process.

Fingers + Feet

When it comes to accessories, some women love shoes, others handbags; me: it's what I like to call finger fashion. From wearing a ridiculous amount of rings all stacked together to elaborate Japanese nail art, the more I can adorn my fingers, the happier I am. Polka dots? Check. Hand-painted flowers? Check. Neon tips, glittered ombré, grommet-encrusted half moons? Check, check, check. Why? Perhaps it's because I spend an enormous amount of time typing furiously at my computer (which I'm sure most of you can relate to!) and looking down at art on my hands makes me smile. Or perhaps it's because I grew up with a mom with manicure-model-like nails, naturally strong, and always perfectly polished. I'm jealous just thinking about it! Very jealous.

Sadly, though, just as I didn't inherit my mom's sea-foam green eyes, high-as-the-sky cheekbones, or beautifully blonde hair (as much as I've tried to achieve it with more bleach and peroxide than I'd like to admit) whatever gene passes down those rock-hard nails skipped me. Instead, my nails are more like my dad's: naturally thin, prone to peeling, quick to chip, and susceptible to splitting. I also have cuticles that seem to want to grow all the way up the entirety of my nail bed.

Whether you want healthier, tougher talons so you can compete with your mom in at least one beauty contest (I can't!) or just want to extend the life of your manicure, this chapter is full of the tips and tricks I've relied on to take me from wishing I could find a way to make gloves trendy year-round to rocking rings and nail art confidently.

Not a polish fan? Don't worry. There's a lot here for you, too! From removing callouses on your feet (I used to joke that the bottom of my feet looked like those of a ninety-year-old woman who had never worn shoes) to taking dry, cracked heels or chapped hands from sandpaper-like to smooth, these are the beauty recipes for hands and feet worth showing off.

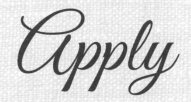

Apply

DIY Beauty Cures for
Fingers + Feet

Yes, a mani/pedi can take your hands and feet from fugly to fab, but you can pamper your fingers and toes at home, too, without the funky chemicals often present in nail salons these days. Whether dry skin, cracked heels, out-of-control cuticles, or discolored nails have you down, these APPLY recipes will make your hands and feet more enviable in no time.

Softening Beer Bath

All skin types

Have leftover beer? Even if it's flat, use it to take your hands and feet from parched to pretty. The yeast in the beer will soften the bottoms of your feet while the alcohol kills bacteria and works as a natural antiseptic. Combined with milk to gently exfoliate and moisturize and honey to hydrate, and this beer bath will give any spa pedicure a run for its money.

8 cups water

1 can beer (any non-light variety)

1 cup whole milk

2 tablespoons raw honey

Heat the water on the stove or use hot water straight from the faucet. You want water to be hot-tub-like hot: comfortably hot, not scorching.

Pour the hot water in a large roasting pan. Add the beer, milk, and honey. Stir until honey is dissolved.

Soak feet in the roasting pan for 10 to 15 minutes.

Follow with Callous Removing Scrub on page 206.

Nail-Whitening Soak

All skin types

Looking for a Crest Whitestrips equivalent for your yellowing nails? Here it is! The sodium bicarbonate in baking soda works to mechanically exfoliate nails of any yellowing residue on your fingers while also helping to brighten and whiten your nails naturally. Baking soda is a mild antiseptic, too, so it will also help prevent infections and control fungus growth, both of which can cause nail discoloration.

2 tablespoons baking soda, divided

6 tablespoons room temperature water, divided

1 teaspoon apricot oil

In each of 2 small bowls, combine 1 tablespoon of the baking soda with 3 tablespoons of the water.

Submerge each clean, polish-free hand in one of the small bowls for 4 to 6 minutes.

Use a nail brush or your fingers to gently rub the mixture over each nail.

Rinse with warm water before massaging nails with the apricot oil.

Quick Tip

• Are you a nail biter? Apply hot sauce to the tips of your nails with a cotton swab and let them dry for a spicy reminder to keep your fingers away from your mouth!

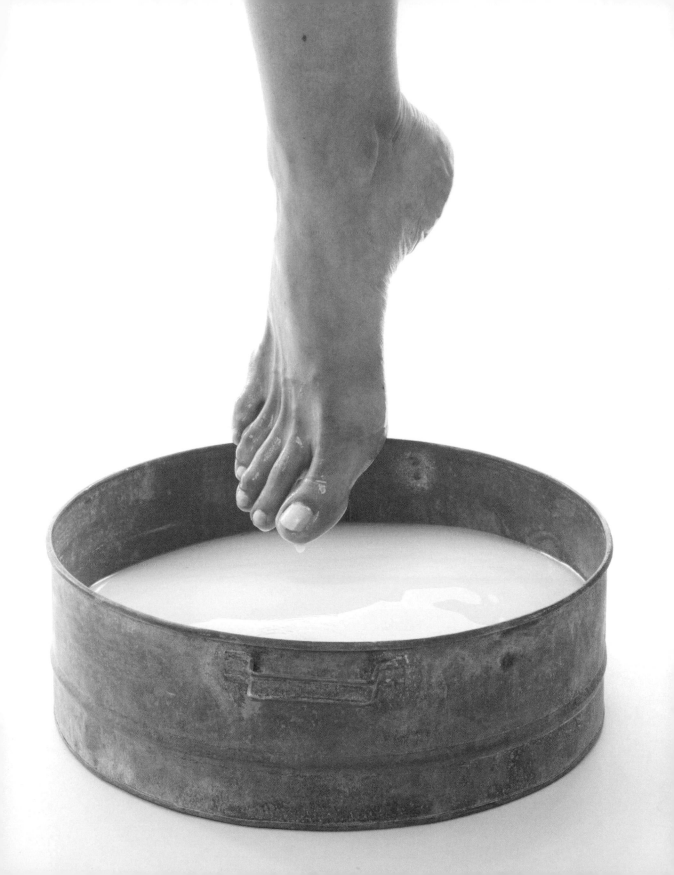

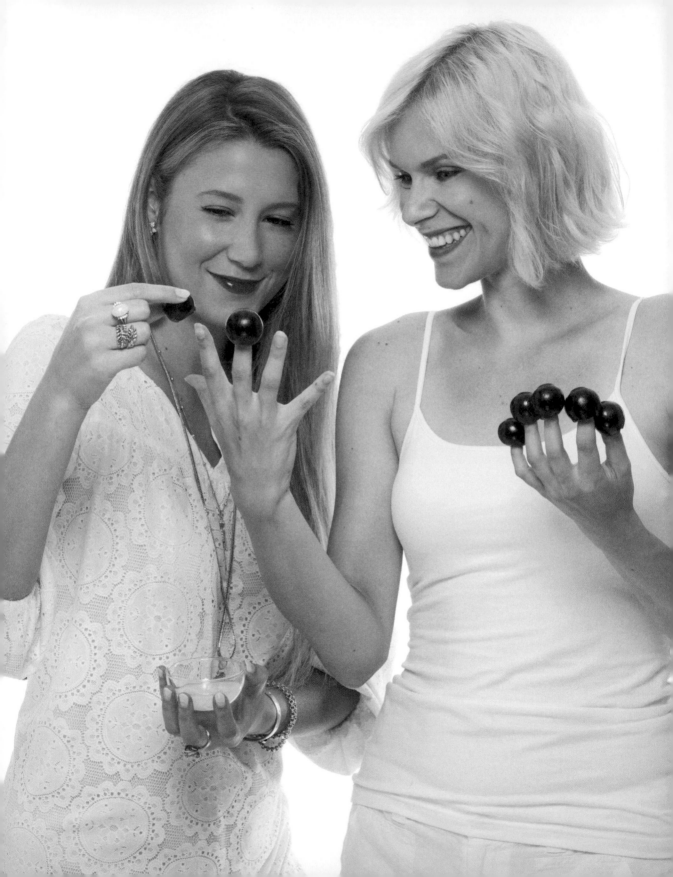

Out-of-Control Cuticles Cure

Not for use on peeling hangnails or open skin

If your cuticles have a life of their own, this is for you. The fruit acids in the grapes gently break down the thin skin around your nails while the white sugar gently scrubs it away. Apricot oil, with a lipid level similar to that of our skin and an especially thin consistency for easy absorption, hydrates dry nails and chapped cuticles naturally. Use this on clean, polish-free fingers for stronger nails and more controlled cuticles.

**1 tablespoon apricot oil
(or apricot seed oil)**
1 tablespoon white sugar
10 large grapes

In a small bowl, mix the apricot oil with the sugar and set aside.

Cut a small amount of the skin off of the stem side of each of the grapes so you can fit a finger inside.

Dig each of your fingers into the flesh of a grape (so it looks like when you used to put olives on each finger before eating them . . . or maybe that was just me!). Let the grapes cover your fingers for 10 minutes before removing and briefly rinsing your fingers under warm water.

Immediately use the oil and sugar mixture to gently massage finger nails and cuticles.

Use a washcloth to wipe away the sugar and excess oil, leaving some oil to penetrate more deeply over time.

If you're a regular nail lacquer wearer, remove polish and do this treatment the night before applying new polish for optimal benefits.

Quick Tips

• The soluble salts in all-natural ginger ale can naturally bleach discolored nails. Soak fingers in a few tablespoons for 10 minutes to brighten nails naturally.

• Before bed, massage your feet with coconut oil and cover them with socks for softer soles come morning.

Hydrating Hand + Foot Mask

All skin types

If winter weather (or excessive hand washing) has your palms parched and tootsies thirsty, apply this hydrating mask to immediately revive them. With vitamin- and antioxidant-dense banana and moisturizing avocado, your skin will be softened, naturally and effectively! Double the recipe to treat both your hands and your feet.

1 ripe banana

½ ripe avocado

In a mixing bowl, use a fork or immersion blender to purée the banana and avocado until smooth.

Apply a thick layer of the mixture to your hands and/or feet and cover with plastic wrap or place into plastic bags. Let it sit for 15 minutes before washing with warm water.

Double the recipe to treat both your hands and feet.

Callous Removing Scrub

Deborah Lippmann, celebrity manicurist

All skin types

Think skipping out on foot care in the winter months is okay because no one is seeing those tootsies of yours? Think again. As celebrity manicurist and nail pro extraordinaire, Deborah Lippmann explains, "You should be exfoliating all-year long, not just in the spring and summer, because if you wait too long you get those cracks in the back of your heels and your feet hurt, and they just don't fit into your shoes right." To keep your feet in smooth order in and out of sandal season, try this homemade scrub Deborah shared with me. It has coconut oil's lauric acid to break down dry, dead skin naturally, olive oil to moisturize, and sea salt to scrub it all away.

¼ cup coarse sea salt

2 tablespoons extra-virgin cold-pressed coconut oil

2 tablespoons extra-virgin olive oil

In a small bowl, combine all of the ingredients.

After a hot shower or after soaking your feet in warm water for 10 minutes, vigorously scrub softened feet with the mixture. Be sure to scrub most aggressively on your heels and the balls of your feet, but don't forget the sides of your feet, between your toes, and your cuticles.

Rinse the salt off with warm water and pat dry so that the oils remain.

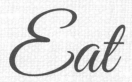

Eat

Food Cures
for Fingers + Feet

Topical beauty recipes may more effectively and immediately tackle acute dry skin, out-of-control cuticles, and discolored nails, but when it comes to getting nails to grow more quickly and considerably stronger, it's all about what you eat.

Ever read the ingredients on a bottle of nail hardening polish? With formaldehyde (the carcinogenic stuff used to preserve dead bodies!) and other gnarly chemicals, most store-bought products designed to give you stronger, longer, healthier nails are pretty gross. Make that *seriously* gross. All hope is not lost, though. Instead of painting chemicals on already weakened nails, let's start at the source and EAT our way to healthier, stronger, and faster growing nails—deliciously.

Maple-Glazed
Coconut Cashews

From Arielle J. Fierman, holistic health coach and chef

Vegetarian, vegan, dairy-free, gluten-free

Could cashews be the key to longer, stronger nails? Yes, yes they can—if you're munching on this maple-glazed variety. High in zinc and healthy fats, cashews help to strengthen and add luster to nails from the inside out. They're prepared with ground flax seeds, which are high in omega-3 fatty acids to reduce inflammation within the nail bed for faster and healthier nail growth. Plus, they're sweetened with maple syrup, which has nail-strengthening vitamin B5, and coconut oil which offers deep moisture.

Serves 8

2 cups raw cashews

⅓ cup maple syrup

2 tablespoons ground flax
   seeds

2 tablespoons dried coconut
   shreds, unsweetened

2 teaspoons extra-virgin
   cold-pressed coconut oil

¼ teaspoon sea salt

In a medium bowl, combine all of the ingredients until the cashews are evenly coated.

Spread mixture evenly on a parchment-lined baking sheet. Broil on high until toasted, approximately 5 minutes, stirring halfway to prevent uneven cooking.

Quick Tips

• Açaí juice is packed with nail-nourishing vitamins. Use it in place of dairy in your next smoothie recipe for added nail-strengthening benefits.

• For severely weak nails, consider adding a biotin supplement to your diet.

Vegetarian Pâté

Vegetarian, gluten-free, dairy-free

When it comes to eating for stronger, healthier nails, protein and iron are where it's at. For vegetarians, getting enough of both can be a challenge—until now. This recipe has eggs and lentils, both of which are protein-packed and iron-rich, plus walnuts for their ample omega-3 fatty acids. This creamy pâté will be just the nutrition your nails need.

Serves 6

1 ¼ cup raw walnuts

1 medium sweet yellow onion, chopped

1 tablespoon olive oil

½ cup mushrooms, chopped

2 cloves garlic, chopped

1 cup canned lentils, drained

4 hardboiled eggs, divided

½ teaspoon salt

1 teaspoon ground black pepper

2 tablespoons fresh parsley, diced

Crackers, to serve

Radishes, thinly sliced, to serve

In a dry skillet, toast the walnuts until fragrant and slightly browned.

Transfer to a food processor and grind it until it's the consistency of chopped liver. Set it aside.

In a large skillet, over low heat, sauté the onions in the oil until softened and they begin to brown. Add the mushrooms and garlic and continue to sauté over low heat until the mushrooms are cooked through and the onions are caramelized, approximately 8 more minutes.

In a food processor, purée the lentils, ¾ of the onion mixture, and 3 of the eggs until combined but still chunky.

Transfer to a mixing bowl and stir in the walnuts, salt, pepper, and remaining onion mixture. Top with remaining egg, diced, and parsley.

Refrigerate to chill and serve with crackers and/or thinly sliced radishes.

Farro + Tuna Salad

From Seamus Mullen, author of *Hero Food* and chef at Tertulia, New York City

With twice the protein of wheat, farro is the nail-bitingly good grain you've been looking for. Served with tuna, which is rich in protein, selenium, and B vitamins for stronger, faster-growing nails, this salad is for nails what fertilizer is for gardens: a key ingredient for healthy growth.

Serves 2

TUNA

2 tablespoons salt

2 tablespoons white sugar

1 teaspoon pimenton (Spanish paprika)

1 lemon, zested

8 ounces fresh tuna

2 cups extra-virgin olive oil

1 orange peel

1 guindilla pepper

2 sprigs thyme

1 clove garlic

FARRO

1 carrot, roughly chopped

½ onion, quartered

1 stalk celery, roughly chopped

1 tablespoon extra-virgin olive oil

1 cup farro

Salt and pepper, to season

1 tablespoon chopped roasted tomato

1 tablespoon chopped castel vetrano olives

1 tablespoon chopped parsley

1 lemon, zested and juiced

1 apple, cored and finely sliced into half moons, to garnish

1 cup frisée, to garnish

For the Tuna

In a mixing bowl, combine the salt, sugar, pimenton, and lemon zest.

Rub all sides of the tuna with the blend and set aside for 15 minutes.

In a medium saucepan, heat the oil over medium heat with the orange peel, pepper, thyme, and garlic, being careful not to let the oil smoke.

Rinse off the tuna and submerge in the warm oil. Cook gently until tuna is just warm in the center and begins to flake. Use a cake tester to check for doneness by inserting the cake tester and then touching it to the inside of your wrist. It should be warm, not hot.

Set it aside to cool to room temperature.

For the Farro

Sauté the carrots, onion, and celery in the oil over medium-high heat until tender.

Add the farro and toast for 1 minute.

Add 4 cups of water and season with the salt and pepper. Bring to a boil and reduce heat to simmer for about 20 minutes.

When the farro is tender, drain it in the colander and remove and discard the carrots, onion, and celery.

Allow the farro to cool to room temperature.

Fold in the tomatoes, olives, parsley, lemon zest, and lemon juice. Fold in the flaked tuna and season with salt and pepper, to taste.

Garnish with the apple slices and frisée.

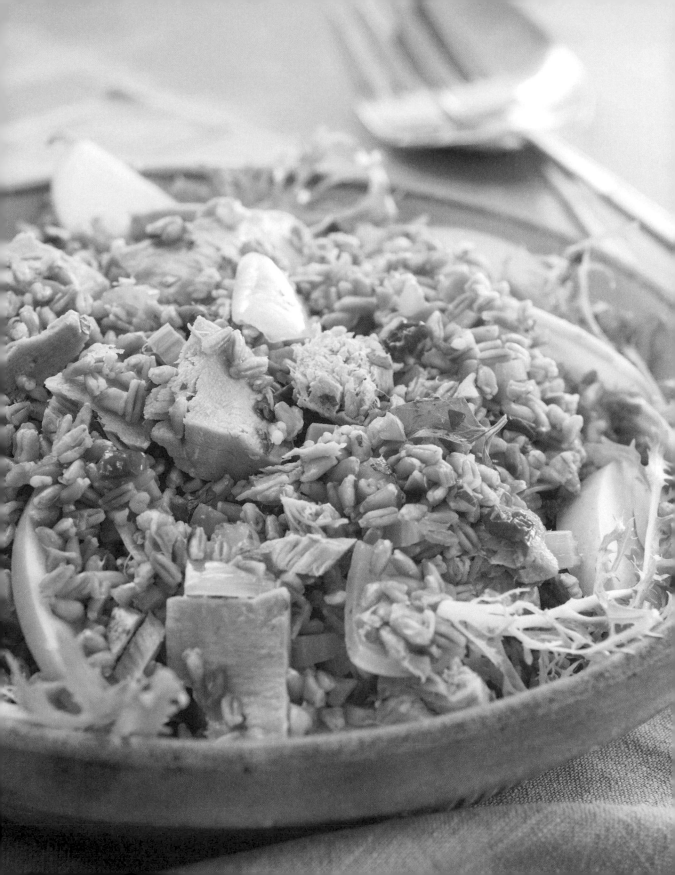

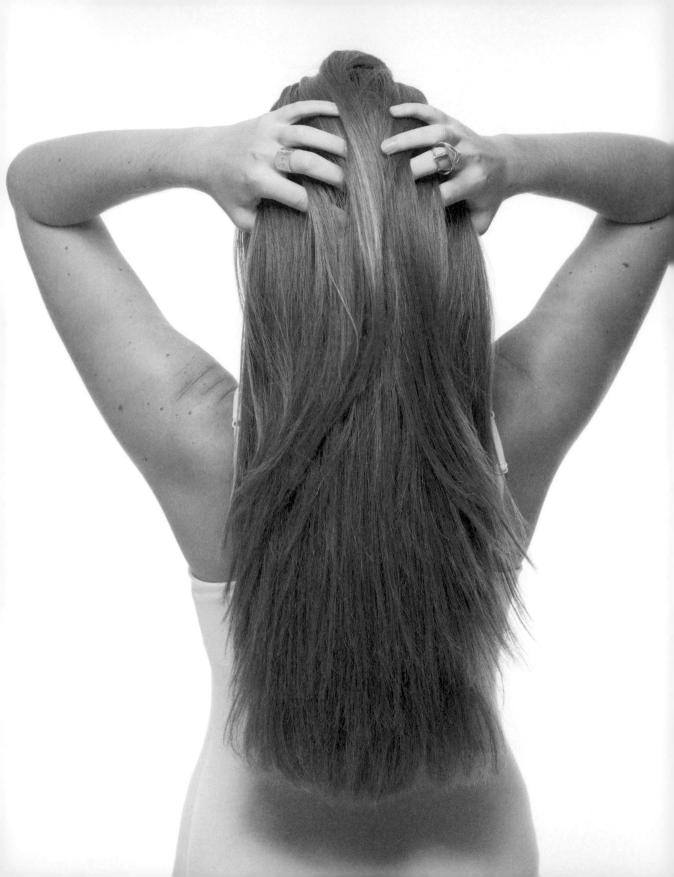

chapter 4
Hair

Thinning, Fine, Slow-Growing Hair

Want to know the first time I became passionate about eating for beauty? When my hair was falling out—literally.

An eating disorder in college (and a bit of a relapse post) left me extraordinarily vitamin-deficient well after my disorder had been resolved (as much as an eating disorder can ever be resolved). My hair was where I most profoundly felt—and saw—the effects of how I had been abusing my body. My formerly luscious locks were breaking and thinning, and not just because of my fondness for hair dye.

There I was, working as a beauty editor. A head full of thinning tresses was not a look I was going for. Practically in tears on the phone at work one day, an intern overheard my situation and told me about tricologist Philip Kingsley. I booked an appointment immediately. While I most definitely expected (hoped for!) a miracle, what I didn't expect was the large focus put on my diet and the foods I needed to load up on to support the health of my precious strands.

Whether your hair has always been thin, is recently thinning, or is just considerably slower to grow in than you would like, both how you treat your hair and your diet work hand in hand to determine the health and beauty of your hair. Today, my hair is long, healthy, and strong. It's not because I've stopped abusing my locks with heat-styling tools and hair dye, but because of how I use food topically and in my diet that my seriously abused strands are as robust as they are.

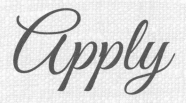

DIY Beauty Cures for Thinning, Fine, Slow-Growing Hair

While abstaining from over processing is the first step to ensuring healthy hair, sometimes steering clear of heat processing and coloring either isn't enough or isn't realistic. Sure, preventing further damage is key, but abstaining from coloring or heat styling your hair isn't the only way to prevent damage. With strengthening, luminizing, volumizing, and nourishing APPLY recipes, you can infuse your hair with the power of food, topically.

Spicy Tequila Scalp Toner

All hair types

Want your hair to grow faster and thicker? Jalapeños have been used in Mexico to encourage hair growth for centuries. Think about how a spicy meal causes your face to flush and your mouth to burn. Similarly, the jalapeño in this spice-fueled hair toner brings blood flow to your scalp, and by increasing circulation, it promotes hair growth. Coupled with the power of tequila, which breaks down product build-up and clears the pores on your head, this toner will ensure your scalp is in prime hair-growing condition.

3 jalapeño peppers, sliced
½ cup tequila

Soak the jalapeño peppers in the tequila overnight (or longer).

Wearing gloves to avoid irritating your hands, use either a saturated cotton pad or an eyedropper to apply the toner to your scalp.

Massage your scalp for 10 minutes before shampooing and conditioning as usual.

Volumizing Hair Rinse

All hair types

If your tresses are fine and limp, beer will do for your hair what it does for your personality—perk it up! The yeast and hops in beer swell the hair shaft and plump the cuticles, for thicker, shinier, and more voluminous strands. Beer's alcohol and acid simultaneously help to break down product build-up. The result: cleaner and thicker hair, naturally. You may smell like a bar, but hey, it's worth it.

1 cup beer, dark brew
1 cup warm water

In a measuring cup or other easy-to-pour container, mix the water and beer.

Apply the mixture to clean, wet hair, using your fingers to ensure even distribution.

Briefly rinse with cool water to lock in the benefits (and dilute the smell!).

Quick Tip
• A scalp massage does more than just feel great; it also helps to stimulate hair growth.

"If your hair lacks body or is extremely fine, pour flat beer into a spray bottle and spritz onto dry hair. Let it air dry and then shower. This adds protein back into the hair, strengthening it and adding body."
   —Edward Tricomi, co-owner of Warren-Tricomi Salons

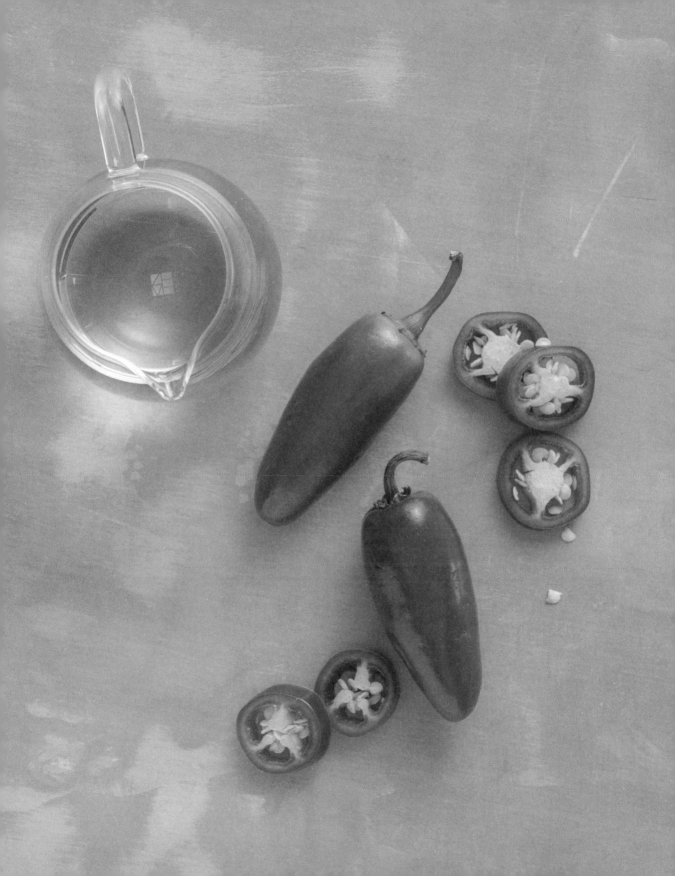

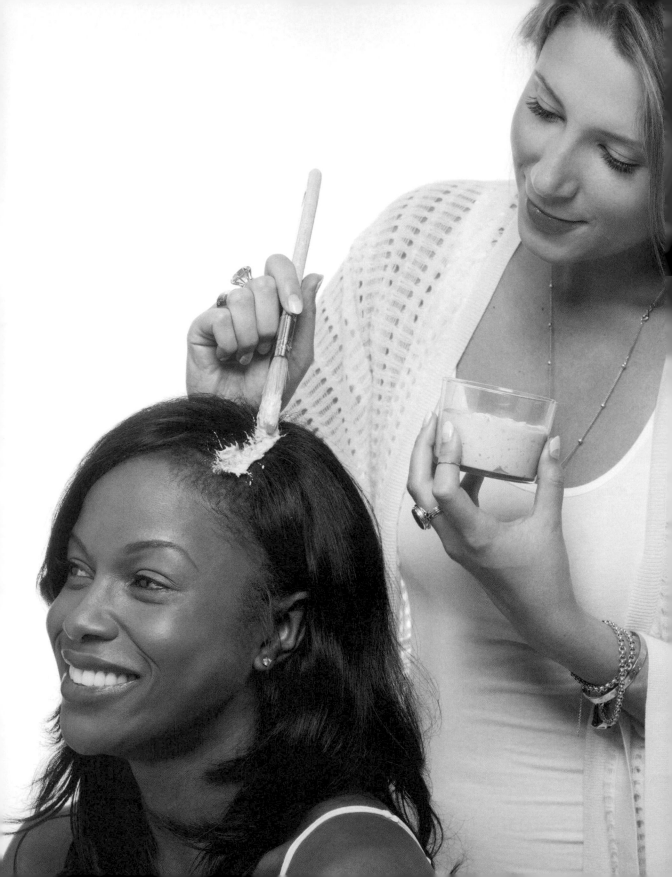

Sour Cream Exfoliating Hair Mask

All hair types (for damaged/color-treated hair, see Note)

A clean, exfoliated scalp is essential for healthy hair growth. Just as clogged pores on your face prevent your skin from breathing properly, clogged pores on your scalp are detrimental to adequate hair growth. With lactic acid and citric acid, in the sour cream and lemon juice, respectively, and with hydrating fats in the avocado, this mask is just what your scalp needs to ensure your hair can grow in healthfully and unencumbered.

½ **ripe avocado**
½ **cup full-fat sour cream**
1 **teaspoon lemon juice**

Using a fork or immersion blender, purée the avocado until smooth.

In a small bowl, combine the avocado with the sour cream and lemon juice.

Apply directly to your scalp, using a wide-tooth comb to section off your hair.

Cover your hair with a shower cap and let it sit for 20 minutes before shampooing and conditioning as usual.

Note: If your hair is extremely dry and damaged or if it's color-treated, leave out the lemon juice for a more gentle scalp exfoliation.

Thinning Hair Booster Tonic

All hair types

This water-based tonic is the perfect rinse-and-go solution for thinning tresses in need of a boost. The thyme in it acts as a scalp stimulant while rosemary encourages hair growth, adds volume, and boosts shine.

2 **cups water**
1 **tablespoon rosemary (dried or fresh)**
1 **tablespoon thyme (dried or fresh)**

Bring the water to a boil.

Remove the water from heat before adding the rosemary and thyme. Cover it and let it sit for at least 1 hour or until cooled to room temperature.

Strain and discard the rosemary and thyme.

Massage the herbal water into your dry (or towel-dried) scalp and hair. Style hair as usual.

Quick Tip
• Condition your hair, not your scalp, to keep the pores on your head clean, healthy, and primed for hair growth.

"You can make a simple hair mask using fresh avocados and olive oil. Massage it into your hair from roots to ends and let it sit for about 20 minutes. Your locks will be so shiny!"
   —Mally Roncal, celebrity makeup artist and founder of Mally Beauty

Eat

Food Cures for Thinning, Fine, Slow-Growing Hair

When your hair is thinning, fine, or slow to grow, just brushing can bring you dangerously close to an anxiety attack. For me, seeing my hair in the brush when I was struggling with thinning hair put me precariously close to a full-blown, I-need-to-breathe-into-a-paper-bag panic attack. Remind yourself that it's normal to lose seventy to one hundred strands of hair each day, and that a panic at what feels like a handful of hair in your brush each morning is only going to increase your stress and hurt your hair health even more. With that in mind, it's time to start eating a hair-healthy diet rich in iron, protein, and B vitamins, all of which a lot of women (especially around that time of the month) are deficient in, and all of which are required for a full head of strong, shiny strands. Since your hair only grows about one-half inch each month, it will take a while for your hair to noticeably improve, but by eating a hair-healthy diet you can prevent further hair loss relatively quickly.

Creamless Creamed Spinach

From Blake Beshore, chef and author of the James Beard Award–winning book
Notes from a Kitchen: A Journey Inside Culinary Obsession
Vegetarian, vegan, dairy-free, gluten-free, nut-free

For a lot of women dealing with fine or slow-growing hair, or even hair loss, an iron deficiency is to blame. Tap into your inner Popeye by loading up on spinach and your hair will thank you! Loaded with folate (needed to create red blood cells) and iron (which helps red blood cells carry oxygen throughout your body), spinach packs a punch for those of us pining for more luscious locks. Spinach is also loaded with lutein, which your body uses to produce sebum, your body's natural hair conditioner. That helps to ensure your hair will grow in as thick, healthy, and strong as possible.

Serves 4

18 ounces baby spinach

2 cloves garlic, minced

½ white onion, minced

4 tablespoons extra-virgin olive oil

¼ cup chardonnay

¼ cup vegetable stock

1 tablespoon apple cider vinegar

Salt and pepper, to taste

Destem and wash the baby spinach. Set aside.

Bring a pot of salted water to a boil and blanche the spinach for 30 to 60 seconds, for softness.

Sauté the garlic and onions in the oil over medium heat until softened and translucent, approximately 3 to 4 minutes.

Strain the spinach and add to the sauté pan with the garlic and onion mixture. Sauté for 1 to 2 minutes, until all ingredients are evenly distributed.

Divide the spinach mixture in half. Leave half in the sauté pan, reducing the heat to low. Put the other half of the spinach in a food processor and pulse, slowly adding the wine, vegetable stock, and vinegar. Add salt and pepper to taste. The ending consistency should resemble a fine purée with a creamy texture.

Add the spinach purée to the sautéing spinach and bring it back up to temperature.

Season with the salt and pepper, to taste, and serve.

Quick Tip
• Protein is the building block of healthy hair. Eat lean meats, poultry, fish, eggs, tofu, and nuts to keep your hair protein-packed.

Sun-Dried Tomato + Basil Breakfast Burrito

Candice Kumai, *Iron Chef America* **judge, author, and TV personality**
Vegetarian, nut-free

Good hair nutrition begins with getting enough protein, especially in the morning when your hair follicles (much like your energy levels) are in need of a morning boost. Few breakfast options (other than liver, perhaps, but who really wants that in the morning?) are better for thinning, fine, or slow-growing hair than eggs. That's because they're packed with protein, and loaded with zinc, selenium, sulfur, and iron, four essential minerals for healthy, lustrous hair.

Serves 6

2 cups diced red potatoes

2 tablespoons extra-virgin olive oil, divided

1 teaspoon sea salt, divided

1 red or yellow onion, chopped

2 eggs + 10 egg whites

2 tablespoons fresh basil, sliced

½ cup oil-packed sun-dried tomatoes, sliced

⅛ teaspoon black pepper

6 whole-wheat tortillas

½ cup feta cheese, crumbled

Preheat the oven to 375°F.

Toss the potatoes with 1 tablespoon oil and ½ teaspoon salt.

On an aluminum foil-lined baking sheet, roast the potatoes for 25 minutes or until fork tender.

In a skillet, sauté the onion in the remaining 1 tablespoon oil until fragrant, approximately 5 minutes.

Whisk the eggs with the additional egg whites.

Add the egg mixture, basil, tomatoes, pepper, and remaining salt to the pan. Cook over medium-low heat until light and fluffy.

Evenly divide the egg mixture between the tortillas. Top with the roasted potatoes and feta cheese before rolling into a burrito shape.

Quick Tip
• Wet hair is three times weaker than dry hair. Only brush or comb your hair when it's dry and you'll save some valuable strands.

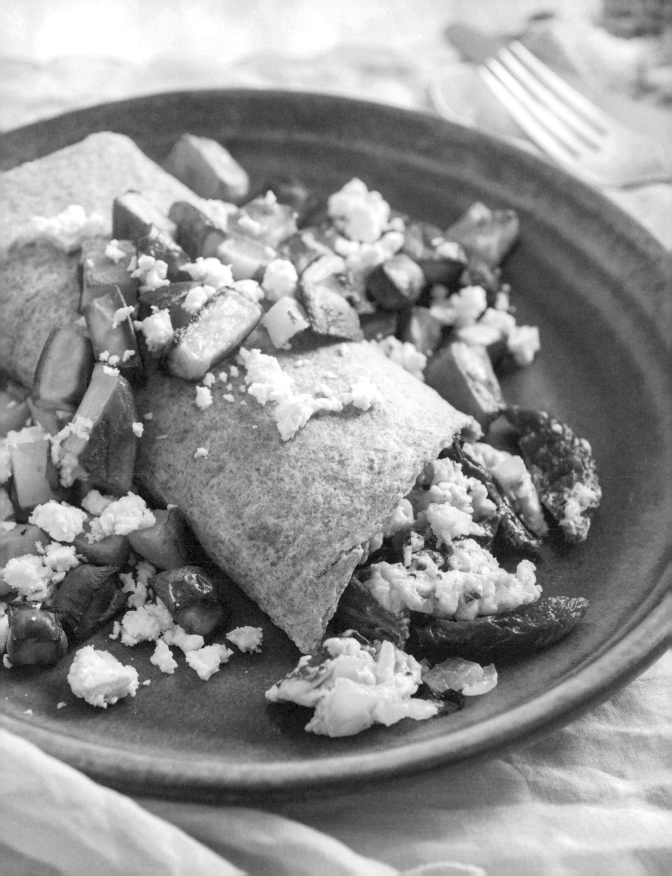

Three-Bean Salad with Shrimp

Dairy-free, gluten-free, nut-free

Beans, beans, they're good for your heart—and your hair! Packed with iron, beans increase circulation, helping your blood carry oxygen throughout your body, including to your scalp. They're also high in protein and iron, which together promote hair growth, help to thicken hair cells, and protect you from anemia-related hair loss. Paired with zinc-rich shrimp, another important mineral for hair growth, this can be your strand-saving salad.

Serves 4

1 pound peeled frozen
   shrimp
2 tablespoons lime juice
3 tablespoons extra-virgin
   olive oil
Salt and pepper, to taste
1 can (15 ounces) black
   beans, drained and rinsed
1 can (15 ounces) kidney
   beans, drained and rinsed
1 can (15 ounces) garbanzo
   beans, drained and rinsed
¼ white onion, diced
¼ cup chopped cilantro
¼ cup chopped parsley
1 jalapeño pepper, seeded
   and minced (optional)
3 small plum tomatoes,
   seeded and chopped
1 avocado, thinly sliced
2 cups brown rice (optional)

Cook the shrimp according to package instructions before cutting them into bite-size pieces.

In a small bowl, whisk together the lime juice, oil, salt, and pepper.

In a large bowl, toss the shrimp with the beans, onion, cilantro, parsley, and jalapeño peppers, if desired.

Chill the bean salad in the refrigerator for several hours to absorb the flavor.

Top the bean salad with the chopped tomatoes and sliced avocado.

Serve over brown rice, if desired.

Quick Tip

• Zinc deficiency can lead to hair loss on your head and eyelashes. Just three ounces of oysters, though, have almost 500 percent of your daily value. So next time you're at a raw bar, slurp up some oysters for more than just their aphrodisiac qualities!

Balsamic Grilled Salmon + Creamy Cranberry Rice

Dairy-free, gluten-free

Complex carbohydrates (like those in brown rice and chickpeas) and protein (like in salmon and beans) are essential for healthy hair growth from the inside out. Also essential: B vitamins and fiber, both of which are ample in this delicious dinner recipe. It's like Rogaine on a plate!

Serves 4

1 cup short-grain brown rice

½ cup raw walnuts

2 ripe avocados, divided

1 cup canned chickpeas, drained and dried

½ cup dried cranberries

½ cup pomegranate seeds

2 teaspoons salt, divided

4 tablespoons high-quality balsamic vinegar, divided

4 fillets salmon (6 ounces)

2 teaspoons olive oil

Salt and pepper, to season

Cook the brown rice according to package instructions. Once cooked, transfer to a large mixing bowl.

Toast the raw walnuts in a dry skillet until slightly brown and fragrant.

In a small bowl, mash 1 of the avocados until creamy.

Stir the mashed avocado into the brown rice until well combined. Toss the toasted walnuts, chickpeas, cranberries, pomegranate seeds, and 1 teaspoon of the salt into the rice. Drizzle with 2 tablespoons of the vinegar and top with the remaining avocado, sliced.

Preheat a grill to medium-high.

Drizzle the salmon with the oil and season with the salt and pepper.

Place the salmon on the grill and cover for 5 to 7 minutes, depending on the thickness of the fish. Flip the salmon and grill for another 4 to 5 minutes.

Drizzle the cooked salmon with the remaining vinegar. Serve with the Creamy Cranberry Rice.

Dry, Dull Hair + Scalp

Lackluster locks may make a splash on a runway every now and then, but dull hair rarely makes it from Fashion Week to work week. Even the models strutting runways or adorning the covers of your monthly glossies with shine-free strands wash the mattifying products out of their hair almost immediately. Here's why: shiny hair is a sign of health and health is always beautiful!

Whether your hair is dry and dull from over-processing, over-drying, or just poor hair health, I have you covered!

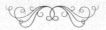

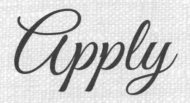

Apply

DIY Beauty Cures
for Dry, Dull Hair + Scalp

Nothing screams health and beauty like a full head of shiny, lustrous locks. Whether you think you pulled the short stick in the genetic lottery or, like me, just never met a bottle of hair-damaging dyes or scorching styling tools you didn't feel compelled to subject your hair to, those lackluster locks are about to be a thing of the past—for good!

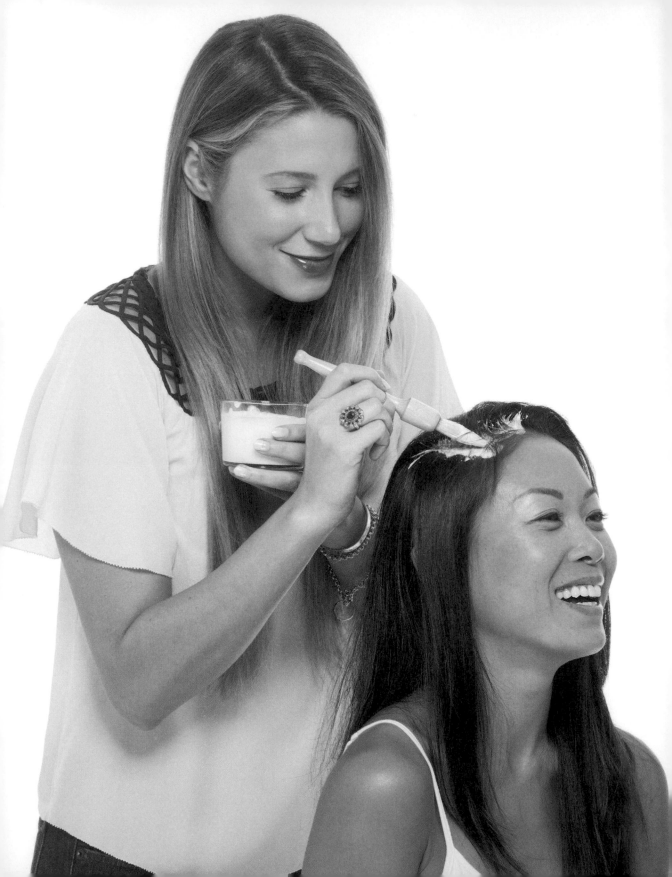

Farewell Flakes Scalp Mask

All hair types

Whether your scalp is dry, itchy, and uncomfortable or just embarrassingly flaky, there's no need to avoid dark clothes for fear of looking like you just walked through a never-melting snowstorm. The key is to exfoliate and moisturize your scalp (and no, an oily head isn't an inevitable by-product of a hydrated scalp). With lactic acid and fat, the sour cream in this dandruff-busting scalp mask helps to dissolve dry, flaking skin and moisturize your scalp, while the cucumber rebalances the water hydration and soothes the discomfort that often accompanies dandruff (as if the flakes weren't enough).

½ cucumber, peeled
½ cup full-fat sour cream

In a blender, purée the cucumber and sour cream until smooth.

Massage the mixture into your hair and scalp. Cover with a shower cap for 30 minutes.

Rinse thoroughly with cool water.

Take It All Off Clarifying Toner

Not for hair damaged from color processing

If your hair's dullness is due to too many products, rather than too much damage, you likely just need to break down the product buildup and shampoo it away. Lucky you! Together, apple cider vinegar and lemon juice break down even the stickiest, greasiest, and most stubborn product buildup. But no matter how much gel, mousse, dry shampoo, and pomade you put on your hair on a daily basis, don't take acid to your hair more than once a week or you'll weaken your hair shaft and invite more serious damage.

If you're using this toner for dandruff, only apply it to your scalp to break down flaky skin cells. Double the recipe if you have very thick or long hair.

3 lemons, juiced
½ cup apple cider vinegar
3 cups warm water

Combine all of the ingredients in a plastic water bottle and shake to combine.

Standing in the shower, slowly pour the mixture on your dry, brushed hair, starting at your scalp and allowing it to run through to the ends of your hair.

When your hair is fully saturated, use your fingers to gently massage the toner into your scalp and through your ends for 3 to 5 minutes.

Do not comb your hair as it will be weakened by the acid.

Shampoo and condition as usual.

Shine-Enhancing Conditioning Treatment

From Porschla Kidd, model

All hair types

When locks are looking lackluster, there's no need to head to the salon for an expensive deep conditioning treatment. Former model Porschla Kidd says, "I always use mayonnaise and eggs for my hair. Mixing 3 to 4 tablespoons of mayo and 2 eggs together makes an amazing conditioner!" With protein, fat, and cholesterol, eggs and mayonnaise combine brilliantly for a highly effective (and cheap!) deep-conditioning treatment you can do at home.

2 eggs

4 tablespoons mayonnaise

Scramble the eggs before mixing with the mayonnaise until well combined.

Apply the mixture to your dry hair from 1 inch away from the scalp to the ends of your hair.

Cover with a shower cap and a hot towel for 15 minutes.

Thoroughly rinse your hair with warm water.

Quick Tips

• Lisa Aharon, lead makeup artist for Kevyn Aucoin, suggests putting coconut oil on your scalp. Part where dry, apply, and let sit as long as you can and rinse out. The lauric acid helps to break down dry skin while hydrating at the same time.

• Champagne isn't just for sipping. Apply equal parts champagne and water to dry hair to enhance shine and brighten natural highlights.

"My favorite DIY beauty tip, as gross as it may seem, is mayonnaise. Just apply mayonnaise to dry hair and leave it on for 25 to 30 minutes, covered with a shower cap. Shampoo really well if you don't want to go out smelling like tuna salad. It'll leave your hair super soft and manageable. Make sure to use the full- fat kind, though. Low-fat mayo just won't cut it!"

—Aly Walansky, ALittleAlytude.com

"I love using apple cider vinegar as a rinse in my hair once a week before I shampoo. It helps to clear any residue off my scalp and product buildup from my hair. It doesn't smell the greatest, but after shampooing, there's no trace of the scent."

—Sarah Conley, StyleITOnline.com

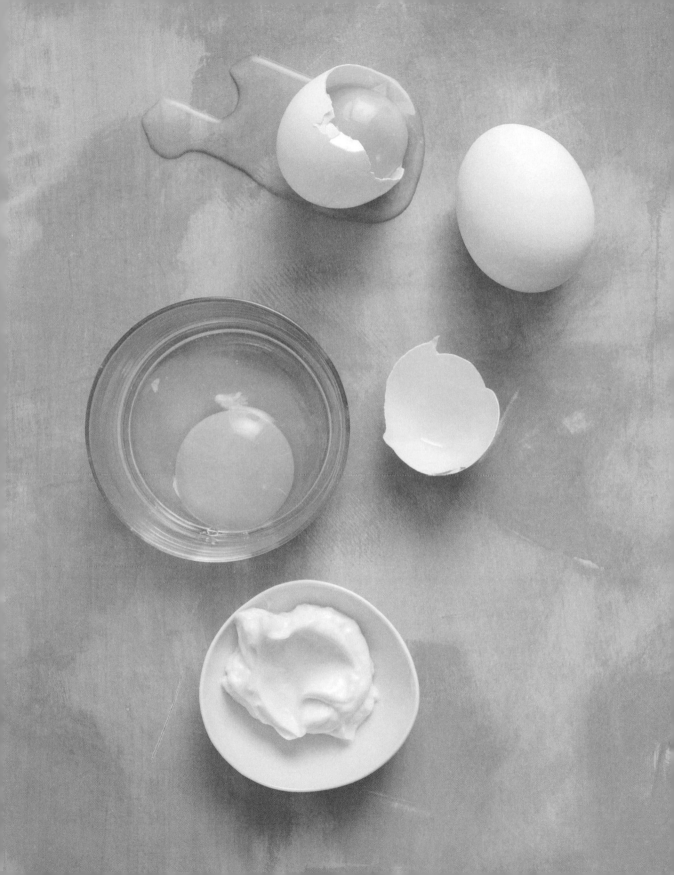

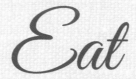

Eat

Food Cures for Dry, Dull Hair + Scalp

Taking locks from lackluster to luminous is about more than applying topical remedies designed to heal and conceal dry, dull hair. It's also about getting to the root cause of your less-than-shiny strands. As your hair's breeding ground, addressing your scalp's health through your diet is the best way to take hair from dehydrated to dynamite, permanently. With these recipes, it's easier (and yummier) than you might think!

Gingered Wild Salmon with Apple Shallot Brandy Glaze

From Dave Martin, chef and *Top Chef* finalist

Gluten-free, nut-free

If your hair and/or scalp are dry, get some fatty fish in your life! It's dense in protein (the building block of your hair) and loaded with omega-3 fatty acids, which are essential for a healthy, hydrated scalp. If you don't like fish you're in luck with this recipe, which was shared with me by chef Dave Martin. Dave says, "I've converted so many people that said they hated salmon until they tried this unique preparation." But for a full head of thick, gorgeous, shiny strands you'd eat just about anything, right? Thankfully, this happens to be Delicious—with a capital *D*.

Serves 2 to 4

GINGERED WILD SALMON

2 tablespoons dry ginger powder

½ cup white sugar

3 tablespoons brown sugar

¼ tablespoon ground nutmeg

3 tablespoons kosher salt

1 tablespoon black pepper

1 pound fresh wild salmon fillet, skin off and filleted

1 to 2 tablespoons extra-virgin olive oil

APPLE SHALLOT BRANDY GLAZE

½ cup minced shallots

1 ½ teaspoons extra-virgin olive oil

½ cup sherry wine

½ cup brandy

6 ounces chicken stock

12 ounces apple cider (fresh if possible)

¼ teaspoon ground cinnamon

¼ teaspoon nutmeg

¼ cup brown sugar

½ teaspoon kosher salt

½ teaspoon ground black pepper

1 tablespoon unsalted butter

For Gingered Wild Salmon

Blend ginger, sugars, nutmeg, salt, and pepper together in a bowl, making sure any chunks are smoothed out in the process.

Preheat a cast iron pan or heavy-bottomed skillet over medium-high heat.

Dredge the salmon filets in the dry rub, ensuring all sides of the fish are coated.

Add the oil to the skillet and cook the salmon in the oil for about 2 minutes on each side, to medium rare, longer if desired.

For Apple Shallot Brandy Glaze

Sauté the shallots in the oil until caramelized. Add the sherry and deglaze until almost dry. Deglaze again with the brandy, until about dry.

Add the chicken stock, apple cider, cinnamon, nutmeg, sugar, salt, and pepper. Bring to a full boil for 10 to 15 minutes.

Remove from heat and add the butter.

Serve warm over the Gingered Wild Salmon.

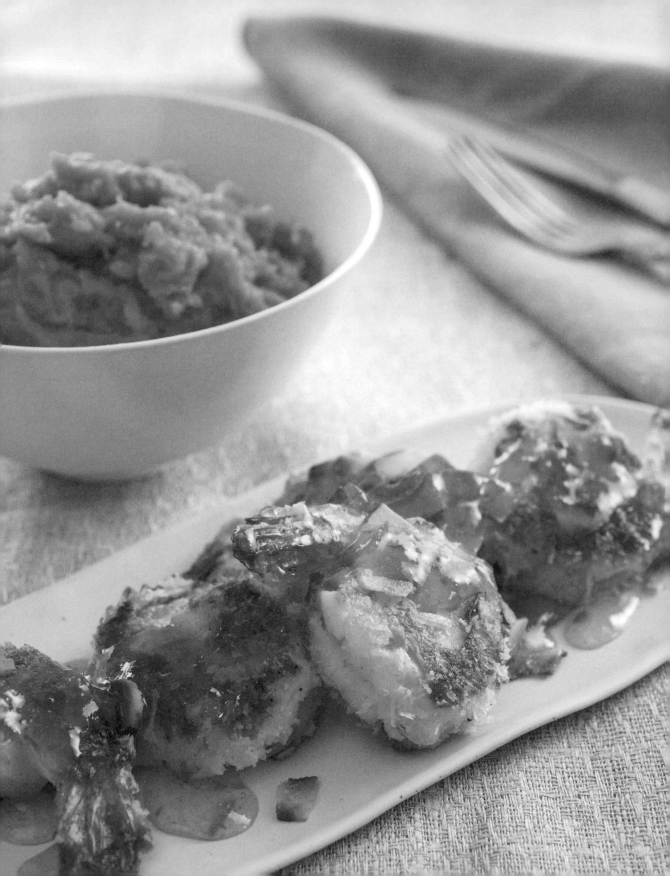

Baked Coconut Shrimp + Sweet Potato Mash with Spicy Marmalade

Dairy-free, nut-free

Mashed sweet potatoes are one of my all-time favorite things to make. Not only because it's so incredibly easy, but also because it's a great way to promote hair health from the inside out. Rich in beta-carotene, which your body converts to skin-saving vitamin A, sweet potatoes help to keep your scalp healthy. Paired with baked shrimp, which are packed with protein, zinc, and copper, this recipe will keep hair growing thick, shiny, and healthy.

Serves 4 to 6

BAKED COCONUT SHRIMP

- ⅓ cup + 3 tablespoons all-purpose flour, divided
- 1 cup unsweetened coconut flakes
- 6 tablespoons panko bread crumbs
- 1 teaspoon salt
- ½ teaspoon ground black pepper
- 3 egg whites
- 1 tablespoon honey
- 1 pound jumbo shrimp (16 to 20 count), peeled (tails left on), deveined
- 2 tablespoons extra-virgin cold-pressed coconut oil

SWEET POTATO MASH

- 2 pounds sweet potatoes, peeled and cubed
- 2 tablespoons extra-virgin cold-pressed coconut oil
- 2 tablespoons coconut milk
- 2 tablespoons fresh squeezed orange juice
- ¼ teaspoon ground cinnamon
- Salt, to taste

SPICY MARMALADE

- ¼ cup orange marmalade
- 2 tablespoons Thai-style chili sauce

For the Baked Coconut Shrimp

Preheat the oven to 450°F.

Put ⅓ cup flour in a small bowl and set aside.

In a shallow bowl, combine the remaining 3 tablespoons flour with the coconut flakes, bread crumbs, salt, and pepper and set aside.

In a separate bowl, beat the egg whites with the honey.

Dredge the shrimp in the flour before dipping them in the egg mixture, letting the excess drip off before pressing the shrimp into the coconut crust mixture, to coat.

In a large skillet, sauté the shrimp in the coconut oil to quickly brown, approximately 30 seconds on each side.

Transfer the shrimp to a pre-greased or non-stick baking sheet in a single layer.

Bake for 8 minutes, flipping halfway through, or until golden on the outside and opaque in the center.

For the Sweet Potato Mash

In a medium pot, boil the sweet potatoes in water until easily pierced with a fork, but not mushy, approximately 20 minutes.

Drain the potatoes and place in a large mixing bowl with the coconut oil, coconut milk, orange juice, and

(continued on next page)

cinnamon. Use a fork, immersion blender, or potato masher to roughly mash the potatoes to your desired consistency. Season with salt, to taste.

For the Spicy Marmalade

In a small bowl, mix the marmalade and chili sauce to combine. Set aside.

Serve the coconut shrimp on top of the sweet potato mash and drizzle with the spicy marmalade.

Quick Tips

• Sleep with a humidifier in your bedroom, which can help your hair retain moisture.

• Washing hair every day can be incredibly drying, so skip a shampoo (or two!) and instead use dry shampoo to absorb excess oil on "off days."

• Steer clear of hair products with lanolin or silicone, which can dry out your hair.

• Think towel drying your hair is best? Think again! Vigorously rubbing your hair with a towel can rough up the cuticle of your hair, leaving it looking lackluster. Instead, gently blot excess water from your hair, avoiding any friction.

• Take colder, shorter showers since hot water can dry you—and your hair!—out.

• Blow-drying your hair? Keep the temperature set to cool to not only protect hair from heat-induced damage but also to keep hair from looking dried out.

Vanilla + Cardamom
Chia Seed Pudding

Vegetarian, vegan, dairy-free, gluten-free

Omega-3 fatty acids aren't just essential for hair and scalp health; they actually make up a percentage of your hair shaft, as well as the membranes in your scalp. Sadly, your body is unable to make those fatty acids on its own, so it's important to make sure you're getting them in your diet. Thankfully, chia seeds are loaded with hair-fertilizing fatty acids. In this vegan pudding recipe, they're combined with almonds for their healing vitamin E; cardamom, long used in ayurvedic medicine to help with a slew of ailments; and walnuts for their shine-inducing biotin and copper.

Serves 2

1 cup raw almonds

2 dates, pitted

1 cup chia seeds, divided

1 teaspoon vanilla extract
  (or 1 vanilla bean, scraped)

1 teaspoon cinnamon

¼ teaspoon cardamom

2 to 4 teaspoons agave,
  to taste

4 tablespoons raw walnuts,
  chopped

Soak the almonds in enough water to cover for at least 8 hours.

Drain the almonds, discarding the water, and transfer them to a high-powered blender. Add the dates and 4 cups of water. Process on high until smooth.

Use a cheesecloth to drain the milk into a mixing bowl. Discard or freeze the "pulp," which you can use in place of flour in other recipes.

Add the chia seeds, vanilla, cinnamon, and cardamom to the milk, stirring until well combined. Refrigerate, uncovered, for at least 90 minutes.

Once fully congealed, stir in agave, as desired, and top with walnuts.

"I'm a huge obsessive kale fan—and Swiss chard. Heavy, hearty greens are antioxidants for your hair. Your hair is constantly being oxidized, but kale and Swiss chard neutralize the chemical compounds. Vidal Sassoon was a huge believer in nutrition for hair, and so am I."

—Michael Forrey, creative director, Vidal Sassoon

Frizz + Other Hair Damage

No shocker here for those of you who know me— or just read my blog on TheBeautyBean.com (which pretty much means you know me)—but my hair is pretty much a never-ending experiment in figuring out just how far I can possibly push it without it breaking, falling out, or just looking like it more aptly belongs on a scarecrow's head. I never met a bottle of hair dye or bleach I didn't immediately want to take to my tresses and I pretty much refuse to let anyone cut my hair unless I'm at least a glass (or three) of champagne in—and I'm not much of a drinker. (What can I say, a traumatizing chop-chop years ago has left me scissor-shy!)

But you would never know it.

If you were to see me taping a TV segment or just on the street, I look like a poster child for hair health, if I do say so myself! (And I don't wear extensions or clip-ins.) The key, for me, is three-fold. First, we need to prevent and counteract the effects of heat styling and coloring. Second, we need to (shhh . . .) fake it—because when you color your hair as much as I do, or even just use a blow-dryer, straightening iron, or curling iron regularly, some amount of hair damage is inevitable. And, thirdly, it's essential to ensure the hair growing in is as healthy as possible. If we're going torture it, we damn well better start with our hair in the best condition possible. The first two we'll tackle in APPLY. The third is all about what we EAT.

Apply

DIY Beauty Cures for Frizz + Other Hair Damage

There's a reason hair care is a $5.9 billion industry in the United States alone. It's because we want thick, shiny, healthy, manageable, frizz-free locks—and we're willing to pay big bucks for it. You, though, don't have to. Instead, head to the kitchen for these practically free DIY beauty recipes for frizz and damage-free locks. Here's a beauty insider's secret: even if you can afford to spend a lot of cash on hair products, the ingredients in your kitchen are often more potent than anything on the shelf in your local beauty supply store. They just don't have the shelf life required to mass-market.

Strand-Saving Sweet Hair Mayonnaise

From Michael Angelo, Wonderland Beauty Parlor, New York City

All hair types

When it comes to my hair, there is no one I trust more than Michael Angelo. I first started seeing him at his Wonderland Beauty Parlor, when after years of over-processing my locks and failing to provide my body (and thus my hair) with adequate nutrients, I had gone back to my natural brunette with the sole intention of preserving the last bit of hair health I still had until I could grow in a healthier head of hair.

I *hated* my natural mousy brown hair. It finally dawned on me that it had to be possible to consistently color your hair and not damage it. Models do it all the time. I just needed to find the person responsible for models' manes and I'd be golden. I called Brooklyn Decker to find out where she went. Her response: Michael Angelo. (Heck, if your parents gave you such an epic name you damn well better live up to it, right?) Needless to say, we fell in love. And my hair is eternally grateful.

The key to a damage-free mane: 1) a colorist who knows what they're doing as well as the limits of your hair. 2) a moisturizing routine to keep your hair as healthy as possible both before and after coloring.

When hair is damaged, your hair shaft, which is supposed to look like a perfect piece of spaghetti, instead looks like a tree trunk that's taken a beating from an axe. With protein-rich egg, hydrating honey and oil, and nutrient-packed banana, this mask will take hair from thin, dry, and damaged, to strong, shiny, and healthy when applied weekly.

1 whole egg

3 tablespoons raw honey

⅓ cup extra-virgin cold-pressed coconut oil

⅓ cup almond oil

⅓ cup avocado oil

1 overripe banana

Place the egg, honey, and 1 tablespoon of water in a food processor, pulsing until well combined.

With the food processor running on low, slowly add the coconut, almond, and avocado oils to the egg mixture until it becomes thick and emulsified.

In a small bowl, mash the banana into a very smooth crème with a fork.

In a mixing bowl, fold the banana crème into the mayonnaise.

Apply the mixture to towel dried, clean hair, using your hands to ensure it's evenly distributed. Cover with plastic wrap for up to an hour.

Shampoo clean and follow with a light detangler.

"As a fitness model, my hair took such a beating from the hot dryers on photo shoots and the sweat at the gym. Now, I'm sure to apply olive oil to the ends of my hair to keep them looking and feeling damage free, all while naturally helping to strengthen my hair."

—Amanda Russell, fitness expert and model

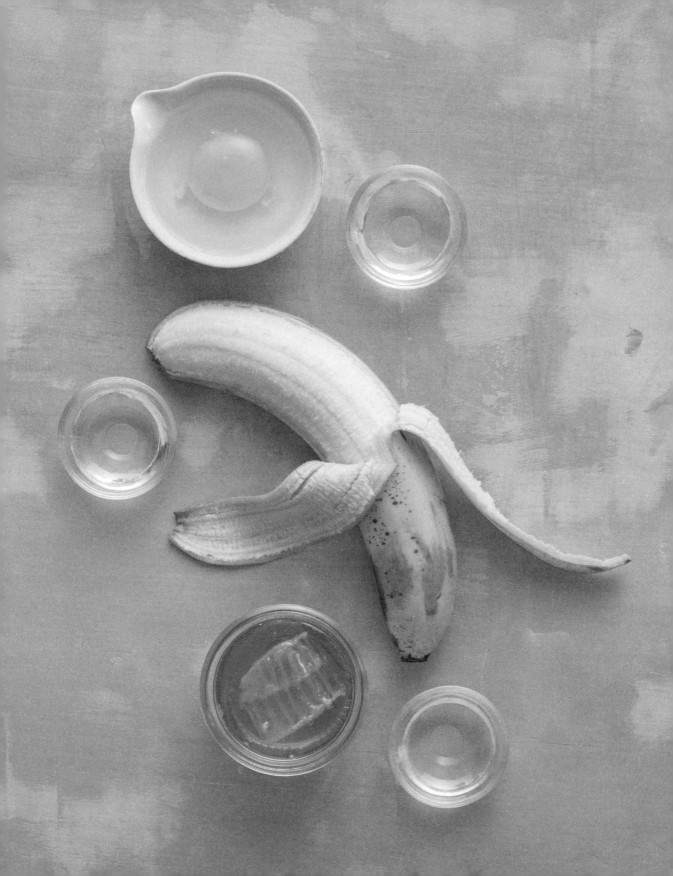

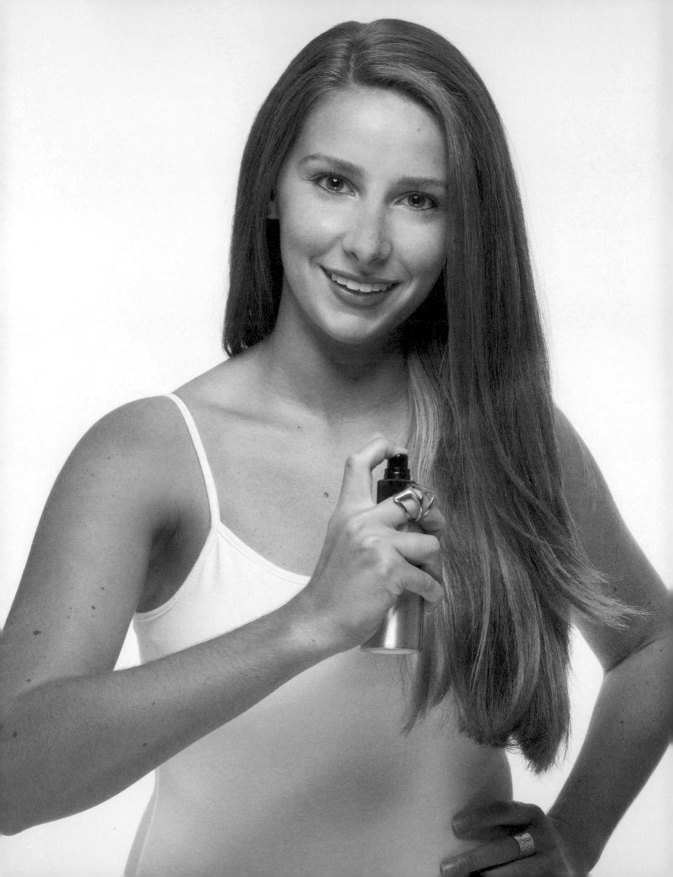

Strand-Saving Beach Spray

All hair types

A day at the beach may be heaven for your mental health, but for your hair, it's more like hell. That warm, comforting sunshine that naturally lightens your locks? It actually severely damages your strands, and the sun-kissed highlights are merely a side effect of the damage. And that's not even mentioning the havoc a day in the salty ocean or a chlorinated pool wreaks on your mane. Just as your body requires a slathering of sunscreen in the summer sun, your hair requires protection from the elements, too. In this spray, antioxidant-packed apricot kernel oil and protective sunflower seed oil hydrate hair and ward off the environmental effects, while filtered water saturates your porous locks so they absorb less salt and chlorine. With this strand-saving beach spray, your hair will stay healthy all summer long.

4 cups filtered, room temperature water
3 tablespoons apricot kernel oil
3 tablespoons sunflower seed oil

In a spray bottle, combine the water and the oils.

Before heading to the beach or pool, shake the bottle to combine the water and the oils before fully saturating your hair with the spray.

Repeat throughout the day, especially before going into the pool or ocean.

Shampoo and condition, as usual, at the end of the day.

Frizz-Fighting Serum

All skin types

Unless you're brushing out tight curls, if you have frizz, it's likely due to damage that's causing your hair to break. Combat frizz once and for all with this leave-in serum. It has avocado oil to fill in the fissures in your hair's cuticle, strengthening your strands against future harm while concealing existing damage; olive oil to improve elasticity; and sweet almond oil to provide UV protection and shine for frizz-free hair from root to tip.

½ cup sweet almond oil
¼ cup avocado oil
¼ cup olive oil

Combine all of the ingredients in a clean spray bottle.

Apply sparingly to dry hair from mid-shaft to ends.

For more controlled application, spray in your hands first before fingering through hair.

For a deeper leave-in treatment, apply liberally before bed and shampoo it out in the morning.

Quick Tip
• Switch to a sulphate-free shampoo for a more moisturized mane. Suds-free shampoo may take getting used to, but it's worth it.

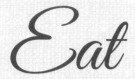

Eat

Food Cures for
Frizz + Other Hair Damage

Your hair may be dead, but that doesn't mean that it's not profoundly affected by how you feed your body. If you've ever had any type of a nutritional deficiency, you likely know that your hair is one of the first places to show the effects of it. By eating for strong, healthy hair, you ensure that the hair that grows in comes out ready to fight damage to the bitter end, even if it's split.

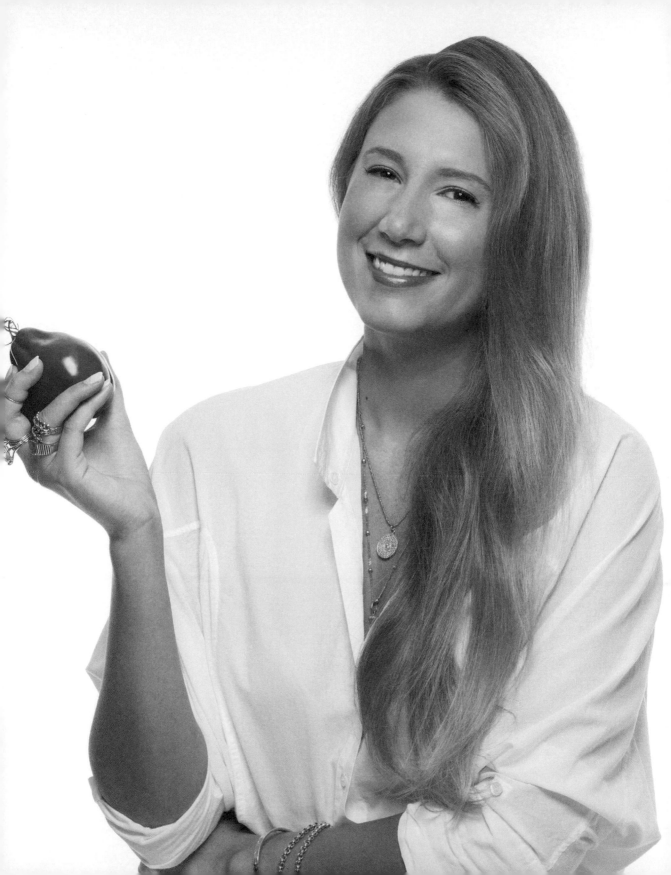

Chinese Five-Spiced Nuts

Vegetarian, dairy-free, gluten-free

Fight frizz and protect your hair from damage with this spiced nut blend that will shield hair from breakage from root to end. With their omega-3 fatty acids, including alpha-linolenic acid, zinc, protein, and healthy fats, the nuts in this blend work together to help condition your scalp and hair from the inside out, for hair more resistant to damage and frizz-causing breakage.

Serves 4 to 8

½ teaspoon Szechwan
  pepper

½ teaspoon ground star anise

¼ teaspoon ground fennel
  seeds

¼ teaspoon ground cloves

¼ teaspoon cinnamon

¼ teaspoon salt

1 egg white

⅓ cup raw honey

½ cup raw walnuts

½ cup raw pecans

½ cup raw almonds

½ cup raw cashews

Preheat the oven to 350°F.

In a small bowl, combine the Szechwan pepper, ground star anise, ground fennel seeds, ground cloves, cinnamon, and salt.

Whisk the egg white with the honey until well combined.

In a mixing bowl, toss the nuts with the egg white and honey mixture. Stir in the dry spices until evenly and thoroughly coated.

Spread the nuts on a parchment-lined baking sheet and bake for 15 to 20 minutes, stirring sporadically to ensure even cooking.

Quick Tip

• Swap your cotton pillowcases, which can snag and break hair, with silk or satin ones to keep breakage at bay.

Eggs + Sweet Potato Hash

Dairy-free, gluten-free, nut-free

This healthy take on a breakfast favorite is made with vitamin A-rich sweet potatoes, which support a healthy scalp primed for optimal hair growth, and iron and protein-packed eggs, which support stronger, shinier, and frizz-free hair. Damage will have nowhere to go but out when you add this decadent-tasting but incredibly healthy recipe to your diet.

Serves 2

2 medium sweet potatoes, peeled

3 tablespoons diced leeks

4 tablespoons extra-virgin olive oil

½ teaspoon salt

½ teaspoon cinnamon

¼ teaspoon black pepper

4 eggs

1 tablespoon diced chives

In a food processor, shred the sweet potatoes.

In a large pan, sauté the leeks in 3 tablespoons of the oil over medium heat, until slightly browned.

Add the sweet potatoes, salt, cinnamon, and pepper and cover for 15 minutes.

Turn flame to high before using a spatula to press the potatoes against the bottom of the pan. Cook until the edges begin to brown, about 5 to 10 additional minutes.

Flip the sweet potato hash and cook for an additional 5 minutes, longer for crispier potatoes.

In a separate pan, heat the remaining tablespoon of oil over medium-low heat. Once hot, crack each of the 4 eggs into the pan. Let cook, uncovered, for approximately 4 minutes so the whites are mostly opaque but the yolks remain runny.

Divide the sweet potato hash between two plates and top each half with 2 sunny-side-up eggs. Garnish with chives.

Quick Tip

- Your hair, like a sponge, can only absorb a finite amount of water. Saturate hair with tap water before hitting the pool or ocean to protect your locks from the damaging effects of chlorine and salt water.

Sardines with Plumped Raisins, Wilted Arugula, + Croutons

From chef Jamie Levine

Dairy-free, nut-free

Packed with healing omega-3 fatty acids, hydrating fats, and strengthening protein, sardines are one of the best foods for hair health. Fret not, though, all of you who fear the canned fish variety. This fresh sardine recipe from chef Jamie Levine is bound to change your mind about sardines.

Serves 4

⅓ **cup raisins**

⅓ **cup concord grape juice**

6 tablespoons extra-virgin olive oil, divided

2 tablespoons thinly sliced scallions (about 8 scallions)

1 clove garlic, minced

3 ounces wild arugula

Kosher salt and pepper, to taste

12 fresh sardine fillets (from 6 fish), skin on

A handful of good quality garlic croutons, crushed into small pieces, to serve

In a small saucepan, bring the raisins and concord grape juice to a simmer. Turn off heat and set aside.

In a large sauté pan, over medium heat, add 2 tablespoons of the oil. When the oil is warm, add the scallions and garlic, sweating until fragrant, about 1 minute. Add the arugula and season with salt and pepper. Gently fold it into the scallions, coating with oil, until wilted but still bright green. Set aside.

Pat each filet dry with a paper towel and season both sides with salt and pepper. In a large sauté pan, add the remaining 4 tablespoons of oil. When hot, add the sardines, skin side down, and sauté until skin appears golden, about 1 minute. Flip the fish over for about 5 seconds.

Spread the wilted arugula evenly across your serving dish. Top with the sardines, flesh side up. Spoon the raisins and juices across the fillets. Sprinkle with crouton pieces.

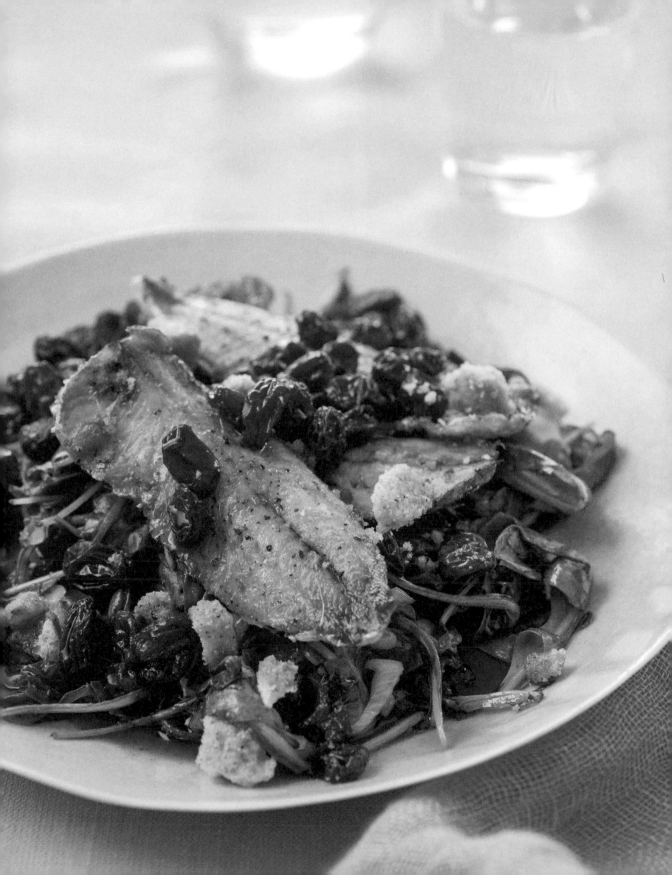

Acknowledgments

Nothing I have ever done has been without the incredible support of the people around me. This book is certainly no exception. A heartfelt thank you far greater than words afford me to . . .

My family—through more tears than I'd like to admit, you have supported me unconditionally, believed in me when I didn't believe in myself, and loved me no matter what. Jeffrey, Stephanie, Teddi, Carly, Lily, Kevin, Andi, Hannah, Ben, Gregg, Cindy, Chase, Madison, and Mackenzie—I can't even begin to thank you for everything. Mom—there aren't enough thank yous in the world to convey just how much I appreciate everything you have done for me. Your grace, strength, and beauty inspire me daily. Dad—thank you not only for being my greatest role model but also for hanging up on me each time I've called you thinking I couldn't accomplish something. You were right. I always could. Together, you have all made me who I am today and for that—and so much more—I am eternally grateful.

Cindy De La Hoz, Corinda Cook, and the entire team at Running Press—thank you for sharing my vision and helping to bring this book to life!

Evan Sung, Eric Bissell, Suzanne Lenzer, Ashely Schleeper, and Maeve Sheridan—your talents are extraordinary! Thank you for sharing your creative brilliance with me.

Michele Martin —you're the best literary agent a girl could have asked for. Thank you for being as excited about this book as I am!

Will Hobbs—from the moment we met (me: in a snood; you: in a suit), I knew I wanted to work with you. Four years later, here we are. Thank you for everything.

Becky Sendrow—even when it would have been easy not to, you stuck in my corner from day one and I will always be extraordinarily grateful for your professional support and personal friendship. You are one in a million.

Amanda Dell—your belief in this book and your connections to the culinary world were invaluable. Thank you for opening up your Rolodex to me—and fact-checking obsessively!

My dream team at WIN PR—especially Jennifer Wilson—you guys are rock stars!

Jen Groover and Karen Salmohnson—just knowing you're in the world makes being an entrepreneur possible.

Desirae Cherman—you are a real beauty—your hair and makeup genius is just icing on the cake.

Aaron Weiss—my only doctor-friend patient enough to answer all my ridiculous (and only tangentially relevant) medical questions. Or just my only doctor friend.

My sisters—Danielle Auerbach, Lauryn Schuman, Julie Burakoff, Katie Herman, and Lacey Stone—without our friendships, I would be lost.

Everyone—past, present, and future—who has worked on or inspired The Beauty Bean including, but certainly not limited to, Alix Turoff, Allison Rapson, Amanda Russell, Arielle Fierman, Ashleigh VanHouten, Becca Gregg, Bianca Beldini, Cady Childs, Caroline Holland, Cate Walker, Chrissy Callahan, Christina Fink, Cindy Augustine, Courtney Leiva, Dayna Brandoff, Diana Zarowin, Elizabeth Monson, Evonne Weiner, Gabrielle Bernstein, Hannah Young, Hillary Rubin, Hitha Palepu, Jacqueline Schwartz, Jenna Nicole Levine, Jennifer Stone, Jessica Bernstein, Jessica Kupetz, Jessie Leventhal, Jill Rudnitzky, Jillian Fleischman, Julia Dzafic, Kaci Kust, Kate Aquillano, Katherine Chen, Kelly Lynn Adams, Kelly McLendon, Kelsea Brennan, Kim Phillips, Kit Rich, Latham Thomas, Lauren Talbot, Laurie Borenstein, Lindsay Danas, Lindsay Tigar, Liz DiAlto, Nicole Teh, Nisha Moodley, Nitika Chopra, Rebecca Alexander, RedBranch PR, Results Advertising, Rosilyn Rayborn, Sabina Ptacin, Sarah Jenks, Sierra Fromberg, Socialyte, and Tayler Bartman.

And, finally, to all the talented chefs who contributed recipes as well as all the celebrities and influencers who shared their beauty secrets, I am extraordinarily appreciative of your willingness to share your beauty recipes with me. Thank you!

Love,
Alexis

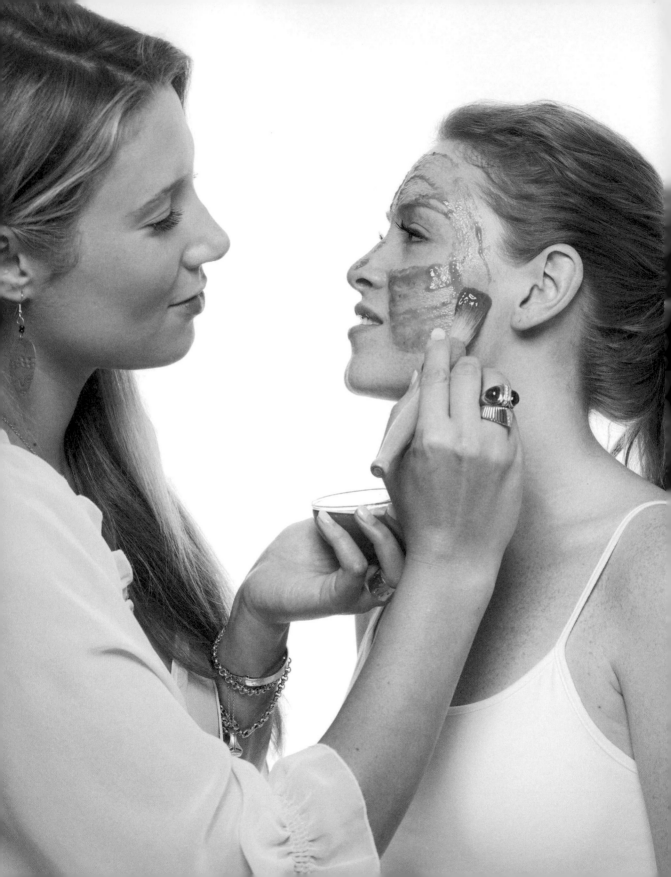

Index

A

açai juice, 208
agave, 64, 105, 171, 197
Age Reversing Wine Mask, 34
allergies, 91, 94, 116
almond butter, 40, 42
Almond Butter + Strawberries, 42
almond milk, 52, 105, 152
almond oil, 240, 243
almonds
    Cereal Crusted Asparagus Fries +
      Yogurt Dipping Sauce, 114, 115
    Chinese Five-Spiced Nuts, 246
    Creamy Butternut Squash Porridge,
      152, 153
    Dukkah-Honey Crusted Halibut, 103
    as exfoliator, 149
    Grilled Nut Butter + Apple Sandwich,
      162, 163
    Olive Oil Granola, 171
    Protein Crackers with Avocado, 81
    Roasted Watermelon Gazpacho,
      128, *129*
    Vanilla + Cardamom Chia Seed
      Pudding, 237
aloe vera juice, 49, 125, 197
anemia, 91
Anti-Acne Apple Astringent, 26
apple cider vinegar, 26, 180, 229, 230
apples
    Donna Karan's Daily Green Juice, 175
    Farro + Tuna Salad, 210, *211*
    Giardino, 151
    Gingered Wild Salmon with Apple
      Shallot Brandy Glaze, 233
    Grilled Nut Butter + Apple Sandwich,
      162, 163
    Nut Butter Chicken Salad Wrap, 51
    Sweet Green Smoothie, 161
    for teeth, 80
apricot oil, 202, 205, 243
arugula, 105, 174, 248
Asian Cabbage Slaw, 29
asparagus, 114
aspirin, 149
avocado
    Avocado, Watercress, + Cumin Salad,
      161
    Avocado + Oatmeal Revival Mask,
      72

    Balsamic Grilled Salmon + Creamy
      Cranberry Rice, 225
    Creamy Kale + Walnut Salad, 94
    Creamy Skin Treatment, 167
    Grilled Salmon Salad, 105
    Hydrating Hand + Foot Mask, 206
    Kale Chips + Spicy Cucumber
      Dip, 172, 173
    Mexicali Rockfish Ceviche, 117
    Piña Colada Polish, 37
    Protein Crackers with Avocado, 81
    Raw Brownie Batter Pudding, 104,
      105
    Raw Green Soup, 78
    Rejuvenating Eye Polish, 100
    Sour Cream Exfoliating Hair Mask, 219
    Strand-Saving Sweet Hair Mayon-
      naise, 240
    Sweet Potato Chips + Cumin Dip, 55
    Three-Bean Salad with Shrimp, 224
    Tropical Crab Salad, 78
Avocado, Watercress, + Cumin Salad, 161
avocado oil, 97, 243

B

Baby Bottom Balm, 167
Baked Coconut Shrimp + Sweet Potato
    Mash with Spicy Marmalade, *234,*
    235–236
baking soda, 146, 202
Balsamic + Goat Cheese Stuffed Figs, 127
Balsamic Grilled Salmon + Creamy Cran-
    berry Rice, 225
banana, 26, 99, 161, 206, 240
basil, 58, 125, 222
Basil Soothing Spray, 125
beans, 224
beef, 151
beer, 202, 216
Beet Salad with Fennel, Orange, + Sun-
    flower Gremolata, 66, 67
berries, 52, 68, 128, 186
beverages
    Donna Karan's Daily Green Juice, 175
    Giardino, 151
    Mint + Ginger Green Tea Lemonade,
      64
    Raw Creamsicle Milk Shake, 139
    Tropical Popeye, 197
Blueberry Crustless Quiche, 186, *187*

Bocconcino di Tartara, 151
Brazil nuts, 40, 163
breakfasts
    Eggs + Sweet Potato Hash, 247
    Garden Vegetable Omelet, 91
    Olive Oil Granola, 171
    Pumpkin Pie Pancakes + Cranberry
      Maple Syrup, 52, 53
    Raw Oatmeal, 30, 31
    Sun-Dried Tomato + Basil Breakfast
      Burrito, 222, 223
broccoli, 91, 116, 130
burrata, 174

C

cabbage, 29
cacao powder, 105
Callous Removing Scrub, 206
Calming + Clearing Milk Mask, 24
Cantaloupe + Carrot Illuminating Mask,
    179
carrots, 28, 91, 142, 161, 179, 210
cashews
    Chinese Five-Spiced Nuts, 246
    Grilled Pineapple with Cashew
      Butter + Vanilla Frozen Yogurt, 188
    Maple-Glazed Coconut Cashews,
      208
    Olive Oil Granola, 171
    Orange Sunshine Soup, 28
    Protein Crackers with Avocado, 81
    Raw Oatmeal, 31
    Turmeric Dip, 197
celery, 51, 142, 151, 161, 175
Cellulite-Concealing Coffee Scrub, 135
Cereal Crusted Asparagus Fries + Yogurt
    Dipping Sauce, 114, *115*
chamomile, 111, 193
champagne, 34, 230
Charred Red Pepper Dip, 183
cheese, 127, 185
chia seeds, 130, 175, 237
chicken, 51, 92, 94
chickpeas, 225
chilies, 54
Chilled Thai Almond Butter Noodles, 40, *41*
Chinese Five-Spiced Nuts, 246
Chopped Veggie Spice Salad, 142
Classic Collard Greens, 131
coconut, 37, 139, 171, 235–236

coconut butter, 197
coconut milk, 197
coconut oil
    Callous Removing Scrub, 206
    Coconut Polish, 136
    for face, 34
    for feet, 205
    for hair, 230
    Lemonade Lightening Scrub, 169
    Milk + Honey Calming Compresses,
        122
    Pre-Shave Oil, 191
    Pumpkin + Coconut Gommage, 76
    Pumpkin Key Lime Brightener, 46
    Raw Oatmeal, 31
    Rejuvenating Scar Scrub, 157
    for shaving, 194
    Strand-Saving Sweet Hair Mayonnaise,
        240
    Two-in-One Anti-Aging Makeup
        Remover, 97
Coconut Polish, 136
coconut water, 139, 197
coffee, 58, 92, 111, 135
Coffee Rubbed Chicken + Farro Salad,
    92, 93
collard greens, 131
Cooling Coffee Compresses, 58
Cooling Cucumber Mask, 125
corn, 91, 117
cottage cheese, 141, 186
cranberries, 52, 171, 225
Cranberry Maple Syrup, 52, 53
cream cheese, 141
Creamless Creamed Spinach, 221
Creamy Butternut Squash Porridge, 152,
    153
Creamy Kale + Walnut Salad, 94
Creamy Salmon Cucumber Boats, 140, 141
Creamy Skin Treatment, 167
Cucumber + Yogurt Cooler, 108
cucumbers
    Baby Bottom Balm, 167
    Chopped Veggie Spice Salad, 142
    Cooling Cucumber Mask, 125
    Creamy Salmon Cucumber Boats,
        140, 141
    Cucumber + Rose Redness Remedy, 61
    Cucumber + Yogurt Cooler, 108
    Donna Karan's Daily Green Juice, 175
    Farewell Flakes Scalp Mask, 229
    Faux-Rested Eye Mask, 89
    Giardino, 151
    Kale Chips + Spicy Cucumber Dip,
        172, 173
    Plump 'Em Up Eye Mask, 99
    Raw Green Soup, 78
    Roasted Watermelon Gazpacho,
        128, 129
    Tropical Crab Salad, 78
Cumin Dip, 55
cumin seeds, 161

Daily Exfoliating Scrub, 194
dates, 31, 237
deserts
    Lemon Berry Parfait, 68, 69
    Raw Brownie Batter Pudding, 105
    Vanilla + Cardamom Chia Seed
        Pudding, 237
Detoxifying Seaweed Bath, 136
dips
    Cereal Crusted Asparagus Fries +
        Yogurt Dipping Sauce, 114, 115
    Charred Red Pepper Dip, 183
    Kale Chips + Spicy Cucumber Dip,
        172, 173
    Sweet Potato Chips + Cumin Dip, 55
    Turmeric Dip, 197
Donna Karan's Daily Green Juice, 175
Dukkah-Honey Crusted Halibut, 103

Egg-cellent Eye Gel, 86
eggs
    Age-Reversing Wine Mask, 34
    Blueberry Crustless Quiche, 186, 187
    Creamy Skin Treatment, 167
    Egg-cellent Eye Gel, 86
    Eggs + Sweet Potato Hash, 247
    for eyes, 99
    Garden Vegetable Omelet, 91
    Gooseberry Meringue Mask, 111
    Hydrating + Blemish-Fighting Facial
        Mask, 23
    Shine-Enhancing Conditioning
        Treatment, 230
    Strand-Saving Sweet Hair Mayonnaise,
        240
    Sun-Dried Tomato + Basil Breakfast
        Burrito, 222, 223
    Vegetarian Pâté, 209
Eggs + Sweet Potato Hash, 247
espresso beans, 92
exercise, 94, 136

Farewell Flakes Scalp Mask, 229
farro, 92, 210, 211
Farro + Tuna Salad, 210, 211
Faux-Rested Eye Mask, 89
fennel, 67, 127, 151, 175
fiber, 31
figs, 127
fish and seafood
    Baked Coconut Shrimp + Sweet Potato
        Mash with Spicy Marmalade, 234,
        235–236

Balsamic Grilled Salmon + Creamy
    Cranberry Rice, 225
Creamy Kale + Walnut Salad, 94
Creamy Salmon Cucumber Boats,
    140, 141
Dukkah-Honey Crusted Halibut, 103
Farro + Tuna Salad, 210, 211
Gingered Wild Salmon with Apple
    Shallot Brandy Glaze, 233
Grilled Salmon Salad, 105
Mexicali Rockfish Ceviche, 117
oysters, 152, 224
Pan-Seared Sea Scallops + Truffled
    Shiitake Rice, 65
Sardines with Plumped Raisins, Wilted
    Arugula, + Croutons, 248, 249
Seared Tuna with Mushroom + Scallion
    "Fried" Brown Rice, 39
Three-Bean Salad with Shrimp, 224
Tropical Crab Salad, 78, 79
flaxseed oil, 117
flaxseeds, 76, 81
frisée, 210
Frizz-Fighting Serum, 243
fruit, dried, 42

Garden Vegetable Omelet, 91
Geisha's Secret Sake Serum, 46
Giardino, 151
ginger, 64, 158, 175, 197, 233
Ginger + Turmeric Massage Oil, 158
ginger ale, 205
Gingered Wild Salmon with Apple Shallot
    Brandy Glaze, 233
Gooseberry Meringue Mask, 111
grape seed extract, 34
grape seed oil, 100, 149, 169
grapes, 37, 51, 72, 205
Green Papaya Salad, 54
Grilled Nut Butter + Apple Sandwich, 162,
    163
Grilled Pineapple with Cashew Butter +
    Vanilla Frozen Yogurt, 188
Grilled Salmon Salad, 105
guava, 180
guava juice, 39
guidelines, 16

ham, 131
hazelnuts, 103, 174
Healing Herbal Tonic, 58
honey, 61
    Almond Butter + Strawberries, 42
    Avocado + Oatmeal Revival Mask,
        72
    Baby Bottom Balm, 167

in bath, 169
Chinese Five-Spiced Nuts, 246
Creamy Skin Treatment, 167
Daily Exfoliating Scrub, 194
Detoxifying Seaweed Bath, 136
Grilled Nut Butter + Apple Sandwich, 162, 163
Honey Glazed Tofu + Orange Broccoli, 116
Hydrating + Blemish-Fighting Facial Mask, 23
for lips, 76
Milk + Honey Calming Compresses, 122
in moisturizer, 72
Nut Butter Chicken Salad Wrap, 51
Optic Tea Treatment, 108
Piña Colada Polish, 37
Plump 'Em Up Eye Mask, 99
Pumpkin + Coconut Gommage, 76
Softening Beer Bath, 202
Strand-Saving Sweet Hair Mayonnaise, 240
Strawberry Clearing Mask, 146
Sweet Lip Scrub, 75
Sweet Potato + Honey Healer, 157
Sweet Watermelon Serum, 122
Tropical Fruit Peel, 24
Wild Strawberries + "Top of the Waldorf Rooftop Honey"-Infused Yogurt, 80
Honey Glazed Tofu + Orange Broccoli, 116
Honey Roasted Delicata Squash Salad, 174
Hydrating + Blemish-Fighting Facial Mask, 23
Hydrating Hand + Foot Mask, 206

Iced Tea Toner, 89
Indian gooseberry juice, 111

jicama, 103

Kabocha Squash with Walnut Pesto, 198, 199
kale, 94, 142, 151, 161, 172, 175, 237
Kale Chips + Spicy Cucumber Dip, 172, 173
kelp, 136
kiwi, 75, 78

leeks, 65, 247
lemon, 68, 146, 151, 161, 169, 229
Lemon Berry Parfait, 68, 69
lemon juice, 46, 49, 157, 179, 180, 219
Lemonade Lightening Scrub, 169
lentils, 209
lettuce, 161, 175
Lightening Overnight Toner, 180
lime, 46, 117, 127
lime juice, 55, 128, 149, 180

mango, 78
maple syrup, 152, 186, 208
Maple-Glazed Coconut Cashews, 208
Margarita Brightening Scrub, 180
marmalade, 235–236
Marmite, 114
mayonnaise, 230
Mediterranean Turkey Burgers, 143
Mexicali Rockfish Ceviche, 117
milk
    Baby Bottom Balm, 167
    in bath, 169
    Calming + Clearing Milk Mask, 24
    Daily Exfoliating Scrub, 194
    Detoxifying Seaweed Bath, 136
    Milk + Honey Calming Compresses, 122
    Rejuvenating Eye Polish, 100
    Rejuvenating Scar Scrub, 157
    Skin Soothing After Shave, 193
    Softening Beer Bath, 202
Milk + Honey Calming Compresses, 122
mint, 26, 64, 76, 80, 188
Mint + Ginger Green Tea Lemonade, 64
mushrooms, 39, 65, 185, 209

Nail-Whitening Soak, 202
Nut Butter Chicken Salad Wrap, 51

oatmeal, 61, 72, 149
oats, 31, 125, 171
olive oil, 72, 76, 149, 169, 191
    Callous Removing Scrub, 206
    Creamless Creamed Spinach, 221
    Frizz-Fighting Serum, 243
    for hair, 219, 240
    Margarita Brightening Scrub, 180
    Olive Oil Granola, 171

onion extract, 158
Optic Tea Treatment, 108
orange, 28, 67, 116, 127, 139
orange juice, 46, 116
Orange Sunshine Soup, 28
Out-of-Control Cuticles Cure, 205

panko breadcrumbs, 114, 235–236
Pan-Seared Sea Scallops + Truffled Shiitake Rice, 65
papaya, 24, 54, 139
parsley, 89
pasta, 130
    Chilled Thai Almond Butter Noodles, 40, 41
    Roasted Broccoli + Sun Dried Tomato Spaghetti, 130
pear, 127, 151
peas, 91
pecans, 171, 246
pepper
    bell, 40, 142, 175, 183
    jalapeño, 216
Perk-Up Potato Packs, 86
pesto, 199
Piña Colada Polish, 37
pine nuts, 199
pineapple, 24, 139, 188, 197
pineapple juice, 37
pistachios, 81, 127, 163, 171
Plump 'Em Up Eye Mask, 99
plums, 92
pomegranate seeds, 174, 225
Portobello Mushroom "Pizza" + Mesclun Greens, 184, 185
potato, 86, 222
Pre-Shave Oil, 191
Protein Crackers with Avocado, 81
pumpkin, 46, 52, 76
Pumpkin + Coconut Gommage, 76
Pumpkin Key Lime Brightener, 46
Pumpkin Pie Pancakes + Cranberry Maple Syrup, 52, 53
pumpkin seeds, 81, 171, 199

raisins, 248
Raw Brownie Batter Pudding, 104, 105
Raw Creamsicle Milk Shake, 139
Raw Green Soup, 78
Raw Oatmeal, 30, 31
Rejuvenating Eye Polish, 100
Rejuvenating Scar Scrub, 157
rice, brown, 39, 65, 224, 225
Roasted Broccoli + Sun-Dried Tomato Spaghetti, 130
Roasted Watermelon Gazpacho, 128, 129

rosemary, 26, 64, 219
roses, 61

S

safflower oil, 191
sage, 58
sake, 46
salads
    Asian Cabbage Slaw, 29
    Avocado, Watercress, + Cumin Salad, 161
    Beet Salad with Fennel, Orange + Sunflower Gremolata, 66, 67
    Chopped Veggie Spice Salad, 142
    Coffee Rubbed Chicken + Farro Salad, 92, 93
    Creamy Kale + Walnut Salad, 94
    Farro + Tuna Salad, 210, 211
    Green Papaya Salad, 54
    Grilled Salmon Salad, 105
    Honey Roasted Delicata Squash Salad, 174
    Lemon Berry Parfait, 68, 69
    Sea Greens Salad, 43
    Shaved Fennel + Blood Orange Salad, 127
    Three-Bean Salad with Shrimp, 224
    Tropical Crab Salad, 78, 79
salt water, 26
sandwiches
    Grilled Nut Butter + Apple Sandwich, 162, 163
    Mediterranean Turkey Burgers, 143
    Nut Butter Chicken Salad Wrap, 51
Sardines with Plumped Raisins, Wilted Arugula, + Croutons, 248, 249
Sea Greens Salad, 43
sea salt, 180, 206
Seared Tuna with Mushroom + Scallion "Fried" Brown Rice, 39
seaweed, 136
sesame seeds, 29, 39, 81, 103
shallots, 233
Shaved Fennel + Blood Orange Salad, 127
Shine-Enhancing Conditioning Treatment, 230
Skin Soothing After Shave, 193
Skin-Lightening Spot Treatment, 49
soba noodles, 40
Softening Beer Bath, 202
sorbet, 68
soups
    Orange Sunshine Soup, 28
    Raw Green Soup, 78
    Roasted Watermelon Gazpacho, 128, 129
sour cream, 167, 219, 229
Sour Cream Exfoliating Hair Mask, 219
soy milk, 49
Special K, 114

Spicy Tequila Scalp Toner, 216
spinach, 142, 161, 175, 186, 197, 221
squash, 152, 174, 199
star anise, 246
starfruit, 149
Starry Spot Treatment, 149
Strand-Saving Beach Spray, 243
Strand-Saving Sweet Hair Mayonnaise, 240
strawberries, 34, 42, 75, 80, 146
Strawberry + Champagne Serum, 34
Strawberry + Kiwi Fruit Peel, 75
Strawberry Clearing Mask, 146
sugar
    brown, 72, 75
    as exfoliator, 72, 76, 149
    raw, 194
    white, 24, 157, 169, 179, 194, 205
Sun-Dried Tomato + Basil Breakfast Burrito, 222, 223
sunflower seeds, 28, 51, 67, 163, 171, 243
Sweet Green Smoothie, 161
Sweet Lip Scrub, 75
Sweet Potato + Honey Healer, 157
Sweet Potato Chips + Cumin Dip, 55
sweet potatoes, 55, 157, 235–236, 247
Sweet Watermelon Serum, 122
Swiss chard, 237

T

tahini, 183
Take It All Off Clarifying Toner, 229
tamanu oil, 158
tea
    black, 89, 108
    chamomile, 111, 193
    green, 37, 64, 111
tea tree oil, 191
tequila, 180, 216
Thinning Hair Booster Tonic, 219
Three-Bean Salad with Shrimp, 224
thyme, 58, 219
tofu, 29, 116
tomatoes, 128, 130, 222
Tropical Crab Salad, 78, 79
Tropical Fruit Peel, 24, 25
Tropical Popeye, 197
turkey, 143
turmeric, 149, 158, 197
Turmeric Dip, 197
Two-in-One Anti-Aging Makeup Remover, 97

V

Vanilla + Cardamom Chia Seed Pudding, 237
Vegemite, 114
Vegetarian Pâté, 209
Volumizing Hair Rinse, 216

W

walnuts
    Balsamic Grilled Salmon + Creamy Cranberry Rice, 225
    Charred Red Pepper Dip, 183
    Chinese Five-Spiced Nuts, 246
    Coffee Rubbed Chicken + Farro Salad, 92, 93
    Creamy Butternut Squash Porridge, 152, 153
    Creamy Kale + Walnut Salad, 94
    Kabocha Squash with Walnut Pesto, 198, 199
    Olive Oil Granola, 171
    Pumpkin + Coconut Gommage, 76
    Raw Brownie Batter Pudding, 104, 105
    Vanilla + Cardamom Chia Seed Pudding, 237
    Vegetarian Pâté, 209
watercress, 161
watermelon, 128, 152
watermelon juice, 122
wheat germ oil, 135, 158
Wild Strawberries + "Top of the Waldorf Rooftop Honey"-Infused Yogurt, 80
wine
    red, 34
    white, 221

Y

yams, 28
yogurt
    Baby Bottom Balm, 167
    Cantaloupe + Carrot Illuminating Mask, 179
    Cereal Crusted Asparagus Fries + Yogurt Dipping Sauce, 114, 115
    Cucumber + Rose Redness Remedy, 61
    Cucumber + Yogurt Cooler, 108
    Faux-Rested Eye Mask, 89
    Grilled Pineapple with Cashew Butter + Vanilla Frozen Yogurt, 188
    Kale Chips + Spicy Cucumber Dip, 172, 173
    Tropical Fruit Peel, 24
    Wild Strawberries + "Top of the Waldorf Rooftop Honey"-Infused Yogurt, 80
    Yogurt + Baking Soda Buffer, 146
Yogurt + Baking Soda Buffer, 146